Polyvictimization

This book provides an overview of the core research and theory on polyvictimization – exposure to multiple types of victimization that may have negative and potentially lifelong biopsychosocial impacts.

The contributors to the volume address such topics as measurement issues in how polyvictimization should be assessed and measured; developmental risks of early childhood polyvictimization for maltreated children in foster care; gender differences in polyvictimization and its consequences among juvenile justice-involved youth; the importance of trauma-focused treatment for polyvictimized youth in the juvenile justice system; and the nature of polyvictimization in the internet era.

Suited to readers who are new to the topic including graduate and under-graduate students, as well as researchers and clinicians who want a concise update on the latest empirical research from the frontiers of this field, this book provides findings and methodological innovations of interest to researchers and human service professionals. This book was originally published as a special issue of the *Journal of Trauma & Dissociation*.

Julian D. Ford is a board certified clinical psychologist, a fellow of the American Psychological Association, and Professor of Psychiatry and Law at the University of Connecticut, USA, where he is Director of the Center for Trauma Recovery and Juvenile Justice and the Center for the Treatment of Developmental Trauma Disorders. He is President of the International Society for Traumatic Stress Studies; and an Associate Editor for the *Journal of Trauma & Dissociation* and *European Journal of Psychotraumatology*. He is the author or editor of 10 books, including *Posttraumatic Stress Disorder* (2009, 2nd Edition), *Treating Complex Trauma: A Sequenced, Relationship-Based Approach* and *Treating Complex Traumatic Stress Disorders in Children* (with Christine Courtois, 2012) and *Adolescents: Scientific Foundations and Therapeutic Models* (with Christine Courtois, 2013).

Brianna C. Delker is Assistant Professor of Psychology at Western Washington University in Bellingham, WA, USA. At Western, Dr. Delker directs the THRIVE Lab (Theory, Healing, and Research on Interpersonal Violence Exposure), serves as a Research Associate at the Center for Cross-Cultural Research, and teaches undergraduate and graduate courses in clinical, developmental, and trauma psychology. She also serves on the Editorial Board of the *Journal of Trauma & Dissociation*.

Polyvictimization

Adverse Impacts in Childhood and
Across the Lifespan

Edited by
Julian D. Ford and Brianna C. Delker

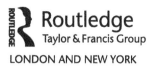

Routledge
Taylor & Francis Group

LONDON AND NEW YORK

First published 2019
by Routledge
2 Park Square, Milton Park, Abingdon, Oxon, OX14 4RN

and by Routledge
605 Third Avenue, New York, NY 10017

First issued in paperback 2020

Routledge is an imprint of the Taylor & Francis Group, an informa business

British Library Cataloguing in Publication Data
A catalogue record for this book is available from the British Library

Typeset in Minion pro
by Newgen Publishing UK

Publisher's Note
The publisher accepts responsibility for any inconsistencies that may have arisen during the
conversion of this book from journal articles to book chapters, namely the inclusion
of journal terminology.

Disclaimer
Every effort has been made to contact copyright holders for their permission to reprint
material in this book. The publishers would be grateful to hear from any copyright holder
who is not here acknowledged and will undertake to rectify any errors or omissions in future
editions of this book.

ISBN 13: 978-0-367-72950-9 (pbk)
ISBN 13: 978-0-367-23546-8 (hbk)

Contents

Citation Information

The chapters in this book were originally published in the *Journal of Trauma & Dissociation*, volume 19, issue 3 (May 2018). When citing this material, please use the original page numbering for each article, as follows:

Chapter 4

Testing gender-differentiated models of the mechanisms linking polyvicti-
mization and youth offending: Numbing and callousness versus dissociation
and borderline traits
Patricia K. Kerig and Crosby A. Modrowski
Journal of Trauma & Dissociation, volume 19, issue 3 (May 2018) pp. 347–361

Chapter 5

When stress becomes the new normal: Alterations in attention and autonomic
reactivity in repeated traumatization
Sarah Herzog, Wendy D'Andrea, Jonathan DePierro, and Vivian Khedari
Journal of Trauma & Dissociation, volume 19, issue 3 (May 2018) pp. 362–381

Chapter 6

Digital poly-victimization: The increasing importance of online crime and har-
assment to the burden of victimization
Sherry Hamby, Zach Blount, Alli Smith, Lisa Jones, Kimberly Mitchell, and
Elizabeth Taylor
Journal of Trauma & Dissociation, volume 19, issue 3 (May 2018) pp. 382–398

For any permission-related enquiries please visit:
www.tandfonline.com/page/help/permissions

Notes on Contributors

Kathryn G. Beauchamp is a Clinical Psychology Intern in Psychiatry and Behavioral Sciences at the University of New Mexico, USA.

Zach Blount is a Post-Baccalaureate Research Fellow at Life Paths Appalachian Research Center, The University of the South, Tennessee, USA.

Ruby Charak is Assistant Professor in the Department of Psychological Science at the University of Texas Rio Grande Valley, USA.

Wendy D'Andrea is Associate Professor of Psychology at the New School, New York City, USA.

Brianna C. Delker is Assistant Professor of Psychology at Western Washington University in Bellingham, WA, USA.

Jonathan DePierro is a Clinical Psychology post-doctoral Fellow at the New York University School of Medicine, USA.

Philip A. Fisher is Professor and Chair of Psychology at the University of Oregon, USA.

Jessica E. Flannery is a doctoral student in the Department of Psychology at the University of Oregon, USA.

Julian D. Ford is Professor of Psychiatry and Law at the University of Connecticut, USA.

Georgina Guilera is Assistant Lecturer in the Department of Behavioural Sciences Methodology at the University of Barcelona, Spain.

Sherry Hamby is Research Professor of Psychology at the University of the South, Tennessee, USA.

Sarah Herzog is a doctoral student in the Department of Psychology (Social Research) at the New School, New York City, USA.

Sarah R. Horn is a doctoral student in the Department of Psychology at the University of Oregon, USA.

Lisa Jones is a research Associate Professor of Psychology at the Crimes against Children Research Center at the University of New Hampshire, USA.

Patricia K. Kerig is Professor of Clinical Psychology at the University of Utah, USA.

Vivian Khedari is studying for a Ph.D. in Clinical Psychology at the New School, New York City, USA.

Kimberley Mitchell is a Research Associate Professor of Psychology at the Crimes against Children Research Center, University of New Hampshire, USA.

Crosby A. Modrowski is a graduate student in clinical psychology at the University of Utah, USA.

Noemí Pereda is a Professor in the Department of Personality, Evaluation and Psychological Treatment at the University of Barcelona, Spain.

Leslie E. Roos is is an Assistant Professor in the Department of Psychology at the University of Manitoba in Winnipeg, Canada.

Anna Segura is Professor of Psychology at the Universitat de Vic, Spain.

Alli Smith is a graduate student in the Department of Psychology at the University of Kansas, USA.

Elizabeth Taylor is a Ph.D. student in the Department of Psychology at Oakland University, USA.

Introduction

Polyvictimization in childhood and its adverse impacts across the lifespan

Julian D. Ford and Brianna C. Delker

ABSTRACT

Although much empirical work has focused on the adverse impact of specific types of childhood victimization (e.g., sexual, physical, or emotional abuse), researchers and clinicians increasingly are recognizing the prevalence of polyvictimization, or exposure to multiple types of victimization. Polyvictimization during formative developmental periods may have detrimental and potentially lifelong biopsychosocial impacts over and above the effects of exposure to specific types of adversity. In this guest editorial, we summarize the key questions and findings for six empirical studies on polyvictimization included in this Special Issue of the Journal of Trauma & Dissociation. These empirical studies further our understanding of the nature, consequences, and assessment of polyvictimization. We conclude with recommendations for continued scientific research and clinical inquiry on polyvictimization.

Although extensive research has focused on the adverse impact of specific types of childhood victimization (e.g., sexual, physical or emotional abuse, and neglect; family and community violence) (D'Andrea, Ford, Stolbach, Spinazzola, & van der Kolk, 2012), researchers and clinicians increasingly have identified particularly high-risk sub-group of children and youth who have been exposed to several *types* of victimization (Finkelhor, Ormrod, & Turner, 2007a). These individuals often continue to experience additional victimization (Finkelhor, Ormrod, & Turner, 2007b), as well as severe and persistent biopsychosocial impairment (Finkelhor, Ormrod, & Turner, 2009; Turner, Shattuck, Finkelhor, & Hamby, 2016). *Polyvictimization* is a term that has been used to describe exposure to multiple types of victimization (Finkelhor et al., 2007a).

Polyvictimization during formative developmental periods (Grasso, Dierkhising, Branson, Ford, & Lee, 2016) may have a severe and potentially lifelong biopsychosocial impact (Andersen, Hughes, Zou, & Wilsnack, 2014; Charak et al., 2016; Hovens, Giltay, Spinhoven, van Hemert, & Penninx, 2015), over and above the effects of exposure to specific types of traumatic stressors and interpersonal adversity (Hamby, Smith, Mitchell, & Turner, 2016). However— and not surprisingly, given the complexity of victimization and related forms of traumatic stressors and adversity—many key questions regarding the nature and impact of polyvictimization remain in need of clarification and fuller answers. In this Special Issue of the *Journal of Trauma and Dissociation*, the results of six empirical studies are reported which help to further our understanding of the nature, consequences, and assessment of polyvictimization. As an introduction to the Special Issue, this commentary will summarize the questions addressed and key findings provided by the six empirical reports. We also will highlight future directions for clinical and scientific investigation and innovation with regard to polyvictimization.

How should polyvictimization be assessed and measured?

Polyvictimization has been operationalized in three principal ways. Over the past two decades, substantial evidence has demonstrated a dose–response relationship between physical and mental health problems and the *cumulative impact* of exposure to an increasing number of types or developmental epochs of victimization (Horan & Widom, 2015; Mustanski, Andrews, & Puckett, 2016; Nilsson, Gustafsson, & Svedin, 2012; Pereda & Gallardo-Pujol, 2014) or adversity (Finkelhor, Shattuck, Turner, & Hamby, 2015; Nurius, Green, Logan-Greene, & Borja, 2015; Ports, Ford, & Merrick, 2015). However, specific types of traumatic exposures also have been shown to account for impairment over and above the cumulative impact of the number of specific exposure types (Grasso et al., 2016; Ports et al., 2015; Wong, Clark, & Marlotte, 2016). A more nuanced approach to identifying the dimensions of traumatic adversity and victimization may be needed in order to determine the contribution of each specific type of adverse exposure, and its interaction with other co-occurring or subsequent types of victimization, in order to fully understand the self-protective adaptations and morbidity/ impairment caused by different profiles of cumulative exposure to trauma and adversity (Ford, 2017; McLaughlin & Sheridan, 2016).

An alternative to the cumulative approach is a categorical perspective that identifies individuals who are classified as polyvictims. This can be done by using a threshold representing whether the extent of exposure to different types of victimization exceeds an *a priori* criterion—either having more types of victimization than average for that sample, i.e., "one-above-the-mean" (Finkelhor et al., 2007a), or a percentile level (i.e., the 90th percentile—the 10% of persons in the sample who experienced the largest number of types of victimization) with some event types (e.g., sexual abuse) weighted higher for adversity (Cyr et al., 2013; Finkelhor et al., 2009; Turner, Finkelhor, & Ormrod, 2010). A second categorical method alternatively identifies mutually exclusive groups of individuals with similar profiles of victimization types using *person-centered* statistical analytic techniques (e.g., latent class analysis; LCA) (Ford, Elhai, Connor, & Frueh, 2010). Polyvictimization also has been identified based on the person's entire childhood (or lifetime), or on recent experiences (typically the past year).

In this issue, Montagut and colleagues describe a study comparing the results of using these three categorical methods of classifying recent and lifetime polyvictims (i.e., the two *a priori* and the *person-centered* methods) with a large school-based sample of adolescents in Spain. Using the well validated Juvenile Victimization Questionnaire, they found that each operational definition and time frame yielded a different set of "polyvictims," with the greatest amount of overlap unexpectedly occurring when the *a priori* one-above-the-mean criterion and the person-centered LCA approach were compared for lifetime polyvictimization, or when the *a priori* top 10% criterion and the LCA approach were compared for past-year polyvictimization. Although the specific youth identified by each approach as polyvictims differed, the demographics (age, gender, socioeconomic status, nationality) of the youth identified as polyvictims were comparable for all the approaches. And, while all of the polyvictims, regardless of how they were identified, tended to have experienced many forms of interpersonal violence, each individual polyvictim's profile of victimization was unique. Lifetime polyvictims were most distinct from other youth in reporting sexual victimization and being assaulted or robbed, while the recent polyvictims tended to most often report victimization by caregivers, siblings, or peers. Thus, different "nets" can be cast to identify polyvictims, and each "net" will identify a different set of youths as polyvictims.

Distinguishing individuals who are classified as polyvictims by several approaches from those who only are identified by only one approach will address several research and clinical questions. For example, it is important to determine both whether the multi-method polyvictims are particularly adversely affected within and across all domains of biopsychosocial functioning. It also is crucial to clinically determine whether individuals who need assistance in preventing or recovering from victimization are being missed when only one of the approaches to identifying polyvictims is used. The findings by Montagut and colleagues also are a vital reminder that no two polyvictims can be assumed to be alike in their individual histories of victimization, let alone in their personal characteristics and the difficulties they face.

How are young children impacted when polyvictimization begins in early childhood?

Infants and toddlers are exposed to traumatic stressors and victimization more often than is commonly assumed (Briggs-Gowan et al., 2010; Briggs-Gowan, Ford, Fraleigh, McCarthy, & Carter, 2010), and they may develop severe biopsychosocial problems including post-traumatic stress disorder (PTSD) (Briggs-Gowan, Carter, & Ford, 2012; Scheeringa, Myers, Putnam, & Zeanah, 2012). Despite the fact that polyvictimization may begin in early childhood, most research and clinical studies on polyvictimization are based on the retrospective report of adults or adolescents on their own (Charak et al., 2016; Grasso et al., 2016; Turner et al., 2016) or (by parents) their child's (Finkelhor, Turner, Shattuck, & Hamby, 2015) childhood history of victimization. In order to confirm those retrospective self- and parent-report findings, it is important to determine whether young children who are polyvictims can be identified based on contemporaneous evidence that is accumulated by an expert source. Although child protective services records are subject to inevitable inaccuracies and biases, they represent a valuable alternative data source for identifying victimized children (Horan & Widom, 2015).

Horn and colleagues collected an immediate and direct assessment of early childhood polyvictimization by extracting Child Protective Services records of maltreatment for toddlers (ages 3–4 years old) in foster care. In addition, they assessed the children's executive function (i.e., cognitive abilities such as memory, processing speed, and verbal abilities), a critical aspect of child development that has been shown to be compromised by exposure to victimization in childhood (Lu et al., 2017) and polyvictimization specifically (Li et al., 2013). Polyvictimized toddlers who had substantial problems with executive function were found to be at heightened risk for clinically significant externalizing (disruptive behavior) problems, while polyvictims with low average or higher executive function skills tended to have at most mild behavior problems. Also, polyvictimization was unrelated to executive function, as well as to the child's age or gender, number of out-of-home placements, and family socioeconomic status.

The findings reported by Horn and colleagues demonstrate that polyvictimization not only has occurred in early childhood for many children who subsequently are placed in foster care, but also that a sub-group of polyvictimized children are at risk developmentally due to deficits in executive function. While the results do not indicate that polyvictimization leads to executive function deficits, they demonstrate that the combination of polyvictimization and executive function deficits can have distinct developmentally adverse effects on behavioral self-control as early as in toddlerhood. This finding is consistent with a meta-model of developmental psychopathology that proposes that distinct trajectories (Briggs-Gowan et al., 2012) must be empirically identified scientifically and clinically in order to characterize the impact of early childhood adversity on the emergence and consolidation of two key domains of biopsychosocial competence: affect regulation and executive functions (Ford, 2005; McLaughlin, 2016).

How does polyvictimization adversely impact high-risk adolescents?

Polyvictimization reaches epidemic levels by the time children grow into adolescence (Ford et al., 2010; McLaughlin et al., 2013). Youth who are troubled and have become involved in the juvenile justice (Cudmore, Cuevas, & Sabina, 2017; Ford, Grasso, Hawke, & Chapman, 2013) and children's mental health (Cuevas, Finkelhor, Ormrod, & Turner, 2009; Ford, Connor, & Hawke, 2009; Ford, Wasser, & Connor, 2011; Segura, Pereda, Guilera, & Abad, 2016) systems are at high risk for polyvictimization. Adolescent polyvictims often have experienced multiple types of victimization in every epoch of development from early childhood through the school years and on into adolescence (Adams et al., 2016; Chan, 2013; Grasso et al., 2016). Polyvictimized adolescents also tend to have particularly severe symptoms of PTSD (Dong, Cao, Cheng, Cui, & Li, 2013; Ford et al., 2010, 2013; Segura et al., 2016; Soler, Paretilla, Kirchner, & Forns, 2012) and dissociation (Leibowitz, Laser, & Burton, 2011; Martinez-Taboas, Canino, Wang, Garcia, & Bravo, 2006; Teicher, Samson, Polcari, & McGreenery, 2006) (Adams et al., 2016; Grasso et al., 2016), It is not clear, however, whether, or how, PTSD and dissociation symptoms play a role in the developmental pathways from polyvictimization to the serious problems with addiction, anger, depression, and suicidality that compromise adolescents' safety and development (Ford et al., 2010)

Ford and colleagues identified three sub-groups in a large sample of juvenile justice-involved youth, including polyvictims, youths with extensive exposure to violence, and youths with histories of mixed adversities including severe accidents, bullying, and the loss of close family members and friends to violent death or suicide. Despite these youths' almost universal exposure to adversity, the polyvictims were found to be uniquely at risk for alcohol/drug use problems compared to their violence- and adversity-exposed peers. Moreover, a stronger relationship was found between PTSD symptoms and problems with anger, depression and anxiety, and somatic/health problems, and between dissociation symptoms and depression, anxiety, and suicidality, for the polyvictims than their violence- and adversity-exposed peers. Thus, youth in the juvenile justice system who are polyvictims not only are at risk for PTSD and dissociative symptoms, but the trauma-related symptoms are particularly likely to contribute to severe and dangerous emotional, behavioral, and self-harm problems for polyvictims. These findings highlight the importance of providing polyvictimized youth who become involved in juvenile justice with trauma-focused treatment that effectively addresses the symptoms of both PTSD and dissociation as well as related safety risks (Ford, Kerig, Desai, & Feierman, 2016).

Girls increasingly are involved in juvenile justice systems, yet the services they receive tend to be no different than those provided to boys (Leve, Chamberlain, & Kim, 2015). As Ford and colleagues, and prior studies (Ford et al., 2013), have shown, girls are substantially over-represented when polyvictim sub-groups are identified among juvenile justice-involved youth (e.g., comprising more than two-thirds of polyvic-tims but less than 20% of the juvenile justice population). Polyvictimized girls are at risk for suicidality (Grigorenko, Sullivan, & Chapman, 2015; Soler, Segura, Kirchner, & Forns, 2013), dissociation (Zona & Milan, 2011), and low levels of perceived self-competence (Soler, Kirchner, Paretilla, & Forns, 2013). Polyvictimized girls also may not experience the protective buffering of being in a stable low-adversity family that appears to protect polyvictimized boys from mental health problems (Nilsson et al., 2012). These findings suggest that polyvictim girls in juvenile justice settings may be at particularly high risk for severe mental health, posttraumatic stress, and dissociative problems.

Therefore, in a mixed-gender sample of juvenile justice-involved youth, Kerig and colleagues investigated the association between gender, polyvicti-mization, emotional numbing and callous unemotional traits, and dissocia-tion and borderline personality traits, with severity of delinquency. Polyvictimization was strongly related to both emotional down-regulation (i.e., numbing and callous unemotional traits) and emotional dysregulation (i.e., dissociation and borderline traits)—and through them, to more severe delinquency—equally for boys and girls. However, the relationships between polyvictimization with delinquency for girls involved two completely inde-pendent paths involving either emotional down-regulation or dysregulation. For boys, however, emotional numbing was associated with emotional dys-regulation (i.e., borderline traits as well as with callous unemotional traits). Thus, polyvictimized girls appear to be at risk for problems with delinquency either due to becoming emotionally shutdown or dysregulated, which may require distinct approaches to treatment and rehabilitation (Chamberlain & Leve, 2004; Chamberlain, Leve, & Degarmo, 2007). The findings also under-score the importance of careful screening for polyvictimization in juvenile justice (Ford et al., 2016), in order to provide interventions for both emo-tional numbing and dissociation before they lead to chronic emotional and behavioral dysregulation that is associated with incarceration and severe behavioral health problems in adulthood (Luntz & Widom, 1994; Lynch et al., 2014; Yanos, Czaja, & Widom, 2010). They also call into question the general stereotype of the delinquent youth as primarily emotionally numbed and callous and unemotional, as well as the gender-specific stereo-type of troubled girls as primarily affectively dysregulated and boys as emotionally shutdown.

Understanding the impact of polyvictimization on the body and mind

The sequelae of traumatic victimization, including PTSD, often involve what at first glance seem to be directly contradictory attentional and behavioral adaptations: on the one hand, hypervigilance to potential threats; yet also an avoidance of contact with or awareness of the settings, situations, or cues that are associated with threat or danger (Ashley, Honzel, Larsen, Justus, & Swick, 2013; Bryant & Harvey, 1997). This apparent paradox has been resolved by postulating an over-arching tendency toward preoccupation with threat—including both attention directed toward and away from cues related to threat—in disorders in which anxiety plays a major role (Pine, 2007).

Herzog and colleagues applied this framework to examine the role of threat-related attention bias in victimization and polyvictimization. Using laboratory tests of attention and physiology (i.e., autonomic nervous system), they found that, in a nonclinical sample of young and mid-life women, those who had experienced a single *type* of interpersonal victimization differed from those who had experienced three or more victimization *types* (i.e., polyvictims). Women who had experienced one type of victimization showed a bias in attention toward threat-related cues (i.e., hypervigilance), while polyvictimized women showed an attention bias away from threat-related cues (i.e., avoidance). In addition, cues associated with relatively mild threats tended to elicit hypervigilance, while cues related to severe threats elicited avoidance. And polyvictims tended to avoid threat cues when their heart rate variability or "vagal tone" (a measure of adaptive regulation of physiological arousal) and heart rate (a measure of the extent of physiological arousal) was low. Thus, a sub-group polyvictims may shift from vigilance to threat cues to avoidance of threat cues in an attempt to modulate even when they experience only relatively mild levels of physiological stress/distress.

These findings suggest that re-victimization may compound the trauma-related coping adaptations that were elicited by earlier experiences of victimization, such that the person who now is a polyvictim may shift from hypervigilance to threat avoidance in an attempt to cope self-protection. This potential shift is strikingly similar to a pattern observed in adults with sub-threshold (i.e., hypervigilance) versus full (i.e., avoidance of threat) PTSD (Thomas, Goegan, Newman, Arndt, & Sears, 2013). Consistent with this view, Herzog and colleagues also found that PTSD symptoms—i.e., stress-related coping involving physiological arousal (Lanius et al., 2010)—were associated with hypervigilance, whereas it was dissociative symptoms—stress reactions that occur when arousal or distress exceed adaptive capacities

(Ford, 2009)—that were related to threat avoidance. Polyvictimization thus may place individuals at risk for complex post-traumatic dysregulation in multiple biological, affective, cognitive, and behavioral domains (Ford, 2013).

Polyvictimization in the Internet era

As technology increasingly permeates not just urban centers but also the traditionally more remote rural places across the globe, victimization has become increasingly technologized and therefore ubiquitous. More than two-thirds of adults in the United States use the Internet (79% of these use Facebook; Greenwood, Perrin, & Duggan, 2016) and nearly three-quarters of teens own a smartphone and use at least one social media website (American Academy of Pediatrics, 2016). Hamby and colleagues take an important first step in addressing the challenges technology poses to our safety and privacy as individuals with a survey of media-based (digital) polyvictimization in a rural population living in southeastern U.S.A. Based on focus groups and qualitative interviews with teens and adults, they identified 11 specific types of digital victimization, including financial scams, hacking, stalking, impersonation, privacy violations, exclusion, and aggression. Almost three in four adults surveyed had experienced at least one of these forms of digital victimization, and consistent with a polyvictimization framework, having a history of in-person victimization doubled the risk of digital victimization. Moreover, digital polyvictimization was equally or more strongly associated with PTSD and anxiety/dysphoria symptoms and problems with health-related quality of life and family well-being than in-person polyvictimization. Study findings suggest that the psychological harm that can be done on the Internet or other media warrants careful assessment and dedicated prevention efforts, as it can be just as severe, or worse, than the harm caused by face-to-face victimization.

Next steps and future directions for studies on polyvictimization

The insights provided by these Special Issue articles attest to the importance of continued scientific research and clinical inquiry concerning the nature and biopsychosocial impact of polyvictimization, beginning in the formative years of childhood (Briggs-Gowan et al., 2010) and adolescence (Grasso et al., 2016), and extending across the lifespan through mid-life and older adulthood (Hamby et al., 2016). Much more clarity is needed as to the different profiles of adversity/victimization that may have distinct outcomes and require correspondingly carefully targeted prevention and therapeutic interventions. The role that specific forms of victimization play in moderating or exacerbating the effects of exposure to differing combinations of multiple types of adversity and victimization requires careful testing.

We also need to better understand the continuities and discontinuities in polyvictimization within and across key developmental epochs and transitions, both for each individual and in the aggregate. The form(s) polyvictimization takes, and the impacts that it has on development and functioning, for populations that are at particular risk for adversity (e.g., people of color, persons of minority sexual identity, homeless persons and families, commercially sexually trafficked youth and adults, immigrants and refugees, developmentally disabled children and adults; people and communities living in poverty or exposed to natural or human-made disasters). These nuances are the translational key to creating targeted interventions (Courtois & Ford, 2009; Ford & Courtois, 2013) enabling polyvictims to recover from traumatic stress, dissociation, and emotion down-regulation and dysregulation while harnessing or developing the resources (Guerra, Ocaranza, & Weinberger, 2016) and "resilience portfolios" (Hamby et al., 2016, p. 217) needed to restore health and self-regulation (Ford, 2013).

The goal of this Special Issue of the *Journal of Trauma and Dissociation* has been to increase awareness of and interest in polyvictimization by clinicians and researchers. We hope this Issue has helped to move this important emerging line of theory, research, and clinical practice toward increasing rigor, consistency, and internal and external validity in defining, conceptualizing, measuring, preventing, and clinically assessing and treating polyvictimization and its sequelae.

Funding

Julian Ford discloses a financial interest as co-owner of Advanced Trauma Solutions, Inc. (ATS), which is licensed by the University of Connecticut to disseminate the TARGET intervention. ATS had no involvement in this article. Brianna Delker has no conflict of interest. Support for writing this article was provided by a grant from the Substance Abuse and Mental Health Services Administration, National Child Traumatic Stress Network, Center for Trauma Recovery and Juvenile Justice (1U79SM080013-01) and Center for the Treatment of Developmental Trauma Disorders (1U79SM080044-01), Julian Ford, Principal Investigator.

References

Adams, Z. W., Moreland, A., Cohen, J. R., Lee, R. C., Hanson, R. F., Danielson, C. K., … Briggs, E. C. (2016). Polyvictimization: Latent profiles and mental health outcomes in a clinical sample of adolescents. *Psychology of Violence, 6*(1), 145–155. doi:10.1037/a0039713

American Academy of Pediatrics. (2016). Why to Limit Your Child's Media Use. Retrieved from https://www.healthychildren.org/English/family-life/Media/Pages/The-Benefits-of-Limiting-TV.aspx

Andersen, J. P., Hughes, T. L., Zou, C., & Wilsnack, S. C. (2014). Lifetime victimization and physical health outcomes among lesbian and heterosexual women. *PLoS One, 9*(7), e101939. doi:10.1371/journal.pone.0101939

Ashley, V., Honzel, N., Larsen, J., Justus, T., & Swick, D. (2013). Attentional bias for trauma-related words: Exaggerated emotional Stroop effect in Afghanistan and Iraq war veterans with PTSD. *BMC Psychiatry, 13*, 86. doi:10.1186/1471-244X-13-86

Briggs-Gowan, M. J., Carter, A. S., Clark, R., Augustyn, M., McCarthy, K. J., & Ford, J. D. (2010). Exposure to potentially traumatic events in early childhood: Differential links to emergent psychopathology. *Journal of Child Psychology and Psychiatry and Allied Disciplines, 51*(10), 1132–1140. doi:10.1111/j.1469-7610.2010.02256.x

Briggs-Gowan, M. J., Carter, A. S., & Ford, J. D. (2012). Parsing the effects violence exposure in early childhood: Modeling developmental pathways. *Journal of Pediatric Psychology, 37* (1), 11–22. doi:10.1093/jpepsy/jsr063

Briggs-Gowan, M. J., Ford, J. D., Fraleigh, L., McCarthy, K., & Carter, A. S. (2010). Prevalence of exposure to potentially traumatic events in a healthy birth cohort of very young children in the northeastern United States. *Journal of Traumatic Stress, 23*(6), 725–733. doi:10.1002/jts.20593

Bryant, R. A., & Harvey, A. G. (1997). Attentional bias in posttraumatic stress disorder. *Journal of Traumatic Stress, 10*(4), 635–644. doi:10.1002/(ISSN)1573-6598

Chamberlain, P., & Leve, L. D. (2004). Female juvenile offenders: Defining an early-onset pathway for delinquency. *Journal of Child & Family Studies, 13*, 439–452. doi:10.1023/B:JCFS.0000044726.07272.b5

Chamberlain, P., Leve, L. D., & Degarmo, D. S. (2007). Multidimensional treatment foster care for girls in the juvenile justice system: 2-year follow-up of a randomized clinical trial. *Journal of Consulting and Clinical Psychology, 75*(1), 187–193. doi:10.1037/0022-006X.75.1.187

Chan, K. L. (2013). Victimization and poly-victimization among school-aged Chinese adolescents: Prevalence and associations with health. *Preventive Medicine, 56*(3–4), 207–210. doi:10.1016/j.ypmed.2012.12.018

Charak, R., Byllesby, B. M., Roley, M. E., Claycomb, M. A., Durham, T. A., Ross, J., … Elhai, J. D. (2016). Latent classes of childhood poly-victimization and associations with suicidal behavior among adult trauma victims: Moderating role of anger. *Child Abuse & Neglect, 62*, 19–28. doi:10.1016/j.chiabu.2016.10.010

Courtois, C. A., & Ford, J. D. (Eds.). (2009). *Treating complex traumatic stress disorders: An evidence-based guide*. New York, NY: Guilford Press.

Cudmore, R. M., Cuevas, C. A., & Sabina, C. (2017). The impact of polyvictimization on delinquency among Latino adolescents: A general strain theory perspective. *Journal of Interpersonal Violence, 32*, 2647–2667. doi:10.1177/0886260515593544

Cuevas, C. A., Finkelhor, D., Ormrod, R., & Turner, H. (2009). Psychiatric diagnosis as a risk marker for victimization in a national sample of children. *Journal of Interpersonal Violence, 24*(4), 636–652. doi:10.1177/0886260508317197

Cyr, K., Chamberland, C., Clement, M. E., Lessard, G., Wemmers, J. A., Collin-Vezina, D., … Damant, D. (2013). Polyvictimization and victimization of children and youth: Results from a populational survey. *Child Abuse & Neglect, 37*(10), 814–820. doi:10.1016/j.chiabu.2013.03.009

D'Andrea, W., Ford, J. D., Stolbach, B., Spinazzola, J., & van der Kolk, B. A. (2012). Understanding interpersonal trauma in children: Why we need a developmentally appropriate trauma diagnosis. *American Journal of Orthopsychiatry, 82*(2), 187–200. doi:10.1111/j.1939-0025.2012.01154.x

Dong, F., Cao, F., Cheng, P., Cui, N., & Li, Y. (2013). Prevalence and associated factors of poly-victimization in Chinese adolescents. *Scandinavian Journal of Psychology, 54*(5), 415–422. doi:10.1111/sjop.12059

Finkelhor, D., Ormrod, R. K., & Turner, H. A. (2007a). Poly-victimization: A neglected component in child victimization. *Child Abuse & Neglect, 31*(1), 7–26. doi:10.1016/j.chiabu.2006.06.008

Finkelhor, D., Ormrod, R. K., & Turner, H. A. (2007b). Re-victimization patterns in a national longitudinal sample of children and youth. *Child Abuse and Neglect, 31*(5), 479–502. doi:10.1016/j.chiabu.2006.03.012

Finkelhor, D., Ormrod, R. K., & Turner, H. A. (2009). Lifetime assessment of poly-victimization in a national sample of children and youth. *Child Abuse & Neglect, 33*, 403–411. doi:10.1016/j.chiabu.2008.09.012

Finkelhor, D., Shattuck, A., Turner, H., & Hamby, S. (2015). A revised inventory of adverse childhood experiences. *Child Abuse & Neglect, 48*, 13–21. doi:10.1016/j.chiabu.2015.07.011

Finkelhor, D., Turner, H. A., Shattuck, A., & Hamby, S. L. (2015). Prevalence of childhood exposure to violence, crime, and abuse: Results from the national survey of children's exposure to violence. *JAMA Pediatrics, 169*(8), 746–754. doi:10.1001/jamapediatrics.2015.0676

Ford, J. D. (2005). Treatment implications of altered neurobiology, affect regulation and information processing following child maltreatment. *Psychiatric Annals, 35*, 410–419. doi:10.3928/00485713-20050501-07

Ford, J. D. (2009). Dissociation in complex posttraumatic stress disorder or disorders of extreme stress not otherwise specified (DESNOS). In P. F. Dell, J. A. O'Neill, & E. Somer (Eds.), *Dissociation and the dissociative disorders: DSM-V and beyond* (pp. 471–485). New York, NY: Routledge.

Ford, J. D. (2013). How can self-regulation enhance our understanding of trauma and dissociation? *Journal ofTrauma and Dissociation, 14*(3), 237–250. doi:10.1080/15299732.2013.769398

Ford, J. D. (2017). Complex trauma and complex PTSD. In J. Cook, S. Gold, & C. Dalenberg (Eds.), *Handbook of trauma psychology* (Vol. 1, pp. 322–349). Washington, DC: American Psychological Association.

Ford, J. D., Connor, D. F., & Hawke, J. (2009). Complex trauma among psychiatrically impaired children: A cross-sectional, chart-review study. *Journal of Clinical Psychiatry, 70*(8), 1155–1163. doi:10.4088/JCP.08m04783

Ford, J. D., & Courtois, C. A. (Eds.). (2013). *Treating complex traumatic stress disorders in children and adolescents: Scientific foundations and therapeutic models.* New York, NY: Guilford.

Ford, J. D., Elhai, J. D., Connor, D. F., & Frueh, B. C. (2010). Poly-victimization and risk of posttraumatic, depressive, and substance use disorders and involvement in delinquency in a national sample of adolescents. *Journal of Adolescent Health, 46*(6), 545–552. doi:10.1016/j.jadohealth.2009.11.212

Ford, J. D., Grasso, D. J., Hawke, J., & Chapman, J. F. (2013). Poly-victimization among juvenile justice-involved youths. *Child Abuse and Neglect, 37*, 788–800. doi:10.1016/j.chiabu.2013.01.005

Ford, J. D., Kerig, P. K., Desai, N., & Feierman, J. (2016). Psychosocial interventions for traumatized youth in the juvenile justice system: Clinical, research, and legal perspectives. *Journal of Juvenile Justice, 5*(1), 31–49.

Ford, J. D., Wasser, T., & Connor, D. F. (2011). Identifying and determining the symptom severity associated with polyvictimization among psychiatrically impaired children in the outpatient setting. *Child Maltreatment, 16*(3), 216–226. doi:10.1177/10775595114061091077559511406109

Grasso, D. J., Dierkhising, C. B., Branson, C. E., Ford, J. D., & Lee, R. (2016). Developmental patterns of adverse childhood experiences and current symptoms and impairment in youth referred for trauma-specific services. *Journal of Abnormal Child Psychology*, *44*(5), 871–886. doi:10.1007/s10802-015-0086-8

Greenwood, S., Perrin, A., & Duggan, M. (2016, November 11). *Social media update 2016: Facebook usage and engagement is on the rise, while adoption of other platforms holds steady*. Retrieved from Pew Research Center http://www.pewinternet.org/2016/11/11/ social-media-update-2016/

Grigorenko, E. L., Sullivan, T., & Chapman, J. (2015). An investigation of gender differences in a representative sample of juveniles detained in Connecticut. *International Journal of Law and Psychiatry*, *38*, 84–91. doi:10.1016/j.ijlp.2015.01.011

Guerra, C., Ocaranza, C., & Weinberger, K. (2016). Searching for social support moderates the relationship between polyvictimization and externalizing symptoms: A brief report. *Journal of Nterpersonal Violence*, 088626051664229. doi:10.1177/0886260516642293

Hamby, S., Smith, A., Mitchell, K., & Turner, H. A. (2016). Poly-victimization and resilience portfolios: Trends in violence research that can enhance the understanding and prevention of elder abuse. *Journal of Elder Abuse and Neglect*, *28*(4–5), 217–234. doi:10.1080/ 08946566.2016.1232182

Horan, J. M., & Widom, C. S. (2015). Cumulative childhood risk and adult functioning in abused and neglected children grown up. *Development and Psychopathology*, *27*(3), 927–941. doi:10.1017/S095457941400090X

Hovens, J. G., Giltay, E. J., Spinhoven, P., van Hemert, A. M., & Penninx, B. W. (2015). Impact of childhood life events and childhood trauma on the onset and recurrence of depressive and anxiety disorders. *Journal of Clinical Psychiatry*, *76*(7), 931–938. doi:10.4088/JCP.14m09135

Lanius, R. A., Vermetten, E., Loewenstein, R. J., Brand, B., Schmahl, C., Bremner, J. D., & Spiegel, D. (2010). Emotion modulation in PTSD: Clinical and neurobiological evidence for a dissociative subtype. *American Journal of Psychiatry*, *167*(6), 640–647. doi:10.1176/ appi.ajp.2009.09081168

Leibowitz, G. S., Laser, J. A., & Burton, D. L. (2011). Exploring the relationships between dissociation, victimization, and juvenile sexual offending. *Journal of Trauma and Dissociation*, *12*(1), 38–52. doi:10.1080/15299732.2010.496143

Leve, L. D., Chamberlain, P., & Kim, H. K. (2015). Risks, outcomes, and evidence-based interventions for girls in the US Juvenile Justice system. *Clinical Child and Family Psychological Review*, *18*(3), 252–279. doi:10.1007/s10567-015-0186-6

Li, Y., Dong, F., Cao, F., Cui, N., Li, J., & Long, Z. (2013). Poly-victimization and executive functions in junior college students. *Scandinavian Journal of Psychology*, *54*(6), 485–492. doi:10.1111/sjop.12083

Lu, S., Pan, F., Gao, W., Wei, Z., Wang, D., Hu, S., ... Li, L. (2017). Neural correlates of childhood trauma with executive function in young healthy adults. *Oncotarget*, *8*(45), 79843–79853. doi:10.18632/oncotarget.20051

Luntz, B. K., & Widom, C. S. (1994). Antisocial personality disorder in abused and neglected children grown up. *American Journal of Psychiatry*, *151*(5), 670–674. doi:10.1176/ ajp.151.5.670

Lynch, S. M., Dehart, D. D., Belknap, J. E., Green, B. L., Dass-Brailsford, P., Johnson, K. A., & Whalley, E. (2014). A multisite study of the prevalence of serious mental illness, PTSD, and substance use disorders of women in jail. *Psychiatric Services*, *65*(5), 670–674. doi:10.1176/ appi.ps.201300172

Martinez-Taboas, A., Canino, G., Wang, M. Q., Garcia, P., & Bravo, M. (2006). Prevalence and victimization correlates of pathological dissociation in a community sample of youths. *Journal of Traumatic Stress, 19*(4), 439–448. doi:10.1002/jts.20144

McLaughlin, K. A. (2016). Future directions in childhood adversity and youth psychopathology. *Journal of Clinical Child and Adolescent Psychology, 45*(3), 361–382. doi:10.1080/15374416.2015.1110823

McLaughlin, K. A., Koenen, K. C., Hill, E. D., Petukhova, M., Sampson, N. A., Zaslavsky, A. M., & Kessler, R. C. (2013). Trauma exposure and posttraumatic stress disorder in a national sample of adolescents. *Journal of the American Academy of Child and Adolescent Psychiatry, 52*(8), 815–830 e814. doi:10.1016/j.jaac.2013.05.011

McLaughlin, K. A., & Sheridan, M. A. (2016). Beyond cumulative risk: A dimensional approach to childhood adversity. *Current Direrctions in Psychological Science, 25*(4), 239–245. doi:10.1177/0963721416655883

Mustanski, B., Andrews, R., & Puckett, J. A. (2016). The effects of cumulative victimization on mental health among Lesbian, Gay, Bisexual, and Transgender adolescents and young adults. *American Journal of Public Health, 106*(3), 527–533. doi:10.2105/AJPH.2015.302976

Nilsson, D. K., Gustafsson, P. E., & Svedin, C. G. (2012). Polytraumatization and trauma symptoms in adolescent boys and girls: Interpersonal and noninterpersonal events and moderating effects of adverse family circumstances. *Journal of Interpersonal Violence, 27*(13), 2645–2664. doi:10.1177/0886260512436386

Nurius, P. S., Green, S., Logan-Greene, P., & Borja, S. (2015). Life course pathways of adverse childhood experiences toward adult psychological well-being: A stress process analysis. *Child Abuse & Neglect, 45*, 143–153. doi:10.1016/j.chiabu.2015.03.008

Pereda, N., & Gallardo-Pujol, D. (2014). One hit makes the difference: The role of polyvictimization in childhood in lifetime revictimization on a southern European sample. *Violence and Victims, 29*(2), 217–231. doi:10.1891/0886-6708.VV-D-12-00061R1

Pine, D. S. (2007). Research review: A neuroscience framework for pediatric anxiety disorders. *Journal of Child Psychology and Psychiatry, 48*(7), 631–648. doi:10.1111/jcpp.2007.48.issue-7

Ports, K. A., Ford, D. C., & Merrick, M. T. (2015). Adverse childhood experiences and sexual victimization in adulthood. *Child Abuse and Neglect, 51*, 313–322. doi:10.1016/j.chiabu.2015.08.017

Scheeringa, M. S., Myers, L., Putnam, F. W., & Zeanah, C. H. (2012). Diagnosing PTSD in early childhood: An empirical assessment of four approaches. *Journal of Traumatic Stress, 25*(4), 359–367. doi:10.1002/jts.21723

Segura, A., Pereda, N., Guilera, G., & Abad, J. (2016). Poly-victimization and psychopathology among Spanish adolescents in residential care. *Child Abuse & Neglect, 55*, 40–51. doi:10.1016/j.chiabu.2016.03.009

Soler, L., Kirchner, T., Paretilla, C., & Forns, M. (2013). Impact of poly-victimization on mental health: The mediator and/or moderator role of self-esteem. *Journal of Interpersonal Violence, 28*(13), 2695–2712. doi:10.1177/0886260513487989

Soler, L., Paretilla, C., Kirchner, T., & Forns, M. (2012). Effects of poly-victimization on self-esteem and post-traumatic stress symptoms in Spanish adolescents. *European Journal of Child and Adolescent Psychiatry, 21*(11), 645–653. doi:10.1007/s00787-012-0301-x

Soler, L., Segura, A., Kirchner, T., & Forns, M. (2013). Polyvictimization and risk for suicidal phenomena in a community sample of Spanish adolescents. *Violence and Victimology, 28*(5), 899–912. doi:10.1891/0886-6708.VV-D-12-00103

Teicher, M. H., Samson, J. A., Polcari, A., & McGreenery, C. E. (2006). Sticks, stones, and hurtful words: Relative effects of various forms of childhood maltreatment. *American Journal of Psychiatry, 163*(6), 993–1000. doi:10.1176/appi.ajp.163.6.993

Thomas, C. L., Goegan, L. D., Newman, K. R., Arndt, J. E., & Sears, C. R. (2013). Attention to threat images in individuals with clinical and subthreshold symptoms of post-traumatic stress disorder. *Journal of Anxiety Disorders, 27*(5), 447–455. doi:10.1016/j.janxdis.2013.05.005

Turner, H. A., Finkelhor, D., & Ormrod, R. (2010). Poly-victimization in a national sample of children and youth. *American Journal of Preventive Medicine, 38*(3), 323–330. doi:10.1016/j.amepre.2009.11.012

Turner, H. A., Shattuck, A., Finkelhor, D., & Hamby, S. (2016). Polyvictimization and youth violence exposure across contexts. *Journal of Adolescent Health, 58*(2), 208–214. doi:10.1016/j.jadohealth.2015.09.021

Wong, C. F., Clark, L. F., & Marlotte, L. (2016). The impact of specific and complex trauma on the mental health of homeless youth. *Journal of Interpersonal Violence, 31*(5), 831–854. doi:10.1177/0886260514556770

Yanos, P. T., Czaja, S. J., & Widom, C. S. (2010). A prospective examination of service use by abused and neglected children followed up into adulthood. *Psychiatric Services, 61*(8), 796–802. doi:10.1176/appi.ps.61.8.796

Zona, K., & Milan, S. (2011). Gender differences in the longitudinal impact of exposure to violence on mental health in urban youth. *Journal of Youth and Adolescence, 40*(12), 1674–1690. doi:10.1007/s10964-011-9649-3

1 Poly-victimization from different methodological approaches using the juvenile victimization questionnaire

Are we identifying the same victims?

Anna Segura, Noemí Pereda, and Georgina Guilera

ABSTRACT

Objective: This study aims to determine whether three different methodological approaches used to assess poly-victimization that apply the Juvenile Victimization Questionnaire (JVQ; Finkelhor, Hamby, Ormrod, & Turner, 2005) identify the same group of adolescent poly-victims. *Method*: The sample consisted of 1,105 adolescents (590 males and 515 females), aged 12–17 years old (*M* = 14.52, *SD* = 1.76) and recruited from seven secondary schools in Spain. The JVQ was used to assess lifetime and past-year experiences of victimization. *Results*: Poly-victims were more likely to experience all types of victimization than victims, regardless of the method used. The degree of agreement between the methods for identifying poly-victimization was moderate for both timeframes, with the highest agreements being recorded between the one-above-the-mean number of victimizations and Latent Class Analysis (LCA) for lifetime, and between the top 10% and LCA for past-year victimization. *Conclusions*: Researchers and clinicians should be aware that the use of different methods to define poly-victimization may mean that different victims are identified. The choice of one method or another may have important implications. In consequence, focusing on how we operationalize poly-victimization should be a priority in the near future.

During the past 15 years, researchers have repeatedly pointed out that interpersonal experiences of violence tend to co-occur across children and adolescents' lives (Turner, Finkelhor, & Ormrod, 2006), meaning that individuals are rarely victims of an isolated type of victimization. Studies have highlighted the importance of assessing a wide range of experiences of violence rather than focusing on a single form (Finkelhor, Ormrod, & Turner, 2007), in order to provide an accurate explanation of child victimization (Hamby & Grych, 2013).

Several frameworks have been designed to analyze this co-occurrence (e.g., multi-type maltreatment, see Higgins & McCabe, 2000; complex trauma, see

Cook et al., 2005; polytraumatization, see Gustafsson, Nilsson, & Svedin, 2009), in attempts to assess the complexity of child and adolescent experiences of violence. Poly-victimization, defined as the experience of multiple types of victimization in different episodes during the course of a child's life (Finkelhor, Ormrod, Turner, & Hamby, 2005), constitutes another framework for addressing this phenomenon, and it seems to affect a high percentage of children and youth across the globe (see Chan, 2013, in China; Cyr et al., 2013, in Canada; Pereda, Guilera, & Abad, 2014, in Spain; Radford, Corral, Bradley, & Fisher, 2013, in the UK). Studies have shown that poly-victimization is higher in countries with lower income levels (Le, Holton, Romero, & Fisher, 2016), but also in children and adolescents at higher risk for victimization, such as sexual minority adolescents (Sterzing, Ratliff, Gartner, McGeough, & Johnson, 2017), adolescents with mental health issues (Álvarez-Lister, Pereda, Abad, Guilera, & the GReVIA, 2014), children cared for by child welfare systems (Cyr et al., 2012) or those involved in the juvenile justice system (Ford, Grasso, Hawke, & Chapman, 2013).

However, few instruments have tried to measure victimization experiences in childhood from a multidimensional, comprehensive perspective that includes different forms of interpersonal violence in different contexts, avoids fragmentation, and acquires the information directly from the children themselves (Hamby & Finkelhor, 2000). Some of these instruments are the Childhood Trauma Questionnaire (CTQ; Bernstein, Ahluvalia, Pogge, & Handelsman, 1997), the ICAST instruments created by the International Society for the Prevention of Child Abuse and Neglect (ISPCAN) (Zolotor et al., 2009), and the Childhood Experiences of Violence Questionnaire (CEVQ) by Walsh, MacMillan, Trocmé, Jamieson, and Boyle (2008). However, these measures focus only on experiences of maltreatment, mainly by caregivers, and therefore do not include all the possible victimization experiences a child may suffer, nor all the contexts in which these incidents may happen (Hamby & Finkelhor, 2000).

Today, most studies addressing the overlap of victimization in children's lives use the poly-victimization approach and apply the Juvenile Victimization Questionnaire (JVQ). For both lifetimes and past-year timeframes, this questionnaire offers a comprehensive assessment of five general areas of child and adolescent victimization: conventional crime, child maltreatment, peer and sibling victimization, sexual victimization, and witnessing/exposure to indirect victimization. The JVQ thus gives a complete profile of child victimization (Finkelhor, Hamby, Ormrod, & Turner, 2005).

However, current methodological methods to the definition of poly-victimization depend on the specific objectives of the research and its time period (i.e., lifetime or past year), the method used (i.e., victims above the mean, the top 10% of child victims, or clustering techniques), the version of the JVQ applied in a particular country (which may include different numbers of items and consider different victimization modules) and the characteristics of the sample (e.g., community, clinical juvenile justice, welfare). All these variables may affect the rates of prevalence recorded. This means that it is difficult to know whether all studies have identified the same at-risk group, namely poly-victims. One of the key aspects in its analysis is the time perspective we apply – that is, over the lifetime, or over the past year. Finkelhor, Ormrod, and Turner (2009) suggested that both lifetime and past-year poly-victimization have advantages and drawbacks. In this regard, they argued that focusing on past-year victimization can guide clinicians towards a more accurate assessment of victimization and can also prevent retrospective biases (Widom, Raphael, & DuMont, 2004); however, a lifetime assessment provides a more complete description of the victimization profile (Finkelhor et al., 2009).

Another key aspect is the approach used to analyze the data. Two approaches have been widely applied to assess lifetime and past year poly-victimization, using three different methods. The first approach sums the variety of victimization experiences lived by a child and focuses on the most victimized adolescents. From this approach, the first method selected children and adolescents who had experienced at least one victimization more than the mean number among the victim group as a whole (Finkelhor et al., 2005). Using this one-above-the-mean method, Finkelhor et al. (2005) considered 22% of the community sample of children interviewed to be past-year poly-victims. For the lifetimeframe, this method has also been applied in some studies, with percentages ranging from 14% to 17% (e.g., Chan, 2013; Dong, Cao, Cheng, Cui, & Li, 2013). Inside the same approach, Finkelhor et al. (2009) proposed another method of identifying poly-victims, consisting in selecting the top 10% of the community sample of children who experienced the highest number of victimizations, both lifetime and past-year. The JVQ lifetime poly-victimization cutoff point for the top 10% of the sample establishes poly-victimization in community samples at more than 11 (Turner, Finkelhor, & Ormrod, 2010), 12 (RadRadford et al., 2013), or 13 different types of victimization (Finkelhor et al., 2009). Finally, the second approach has used clustering methods such as traditional cluster analysis with community and high-risk samples (Álvarez-Lister et al., 2014; Holt, Finkelhor, & Kaufman, 2007) or latent class analysis (LCA) (Kretschmar, Tossone, Butcher, & Flannery, 2016; Reid & Sullivan, 2009; Turner, Shattuck, Finkelhor, & Hamby, 2016). The authors used the responses to the JVQ items (yes/no) as observed categorical variables to identify subgroups of victims with different victimization profiles or combinations of victimization experiences (i.e., clusters or latent classes), among which one or more groups of poly-victims are identified. Using clustering methods, the authors identified the groups who report a high mean of multiple types of victimization experiences as poly-victims.

The present study

Today, researchers apply a range of methodologies to identify the most victimized children and adolescents. This variety may prevent us from consistently selecting the same group of poly-victims across studies. The present study aims to identify poly-victims by applying the different approaches already used in previous studies, and then by examining whether these methods classify the same group of adolescents.

Method

Participants

The sample included 1,105 adolescents (590 males and 515 females) from 12 to 17 years old (M = 14.52 years, SD = 1.76) from Catalonia, the northeastern region of Spain. The inclusion criteria were age between 12 and 17 years old, sufficient cognitive and linguistic abilities to understand the questions in the questionnaire, and willingness to participate. Based on an adaptation of the Hollingshead Four-Factor Index (Hollingshead, 1975) the socioeconomic status of the children's families was as follows: low (1.4%), medium-low (6.2%), medium (12.2%), medium-high (31.8%), and high level (38.4%). This information was not available for 10% of the sample. The majority (94.9%) of the adolescents were born in Spain. Males and females were comparable in terms of age and socioeconomic status. However, male and female participants differed significantly (χ^2 = 4.751, p = .029, OR = 1.829, 95% CI [1.05, 3.17]) in terms of their country of birth (classified as Spain vs. another country).

Procedure

The study has a cross-sectional design. Both parents and youths were informed of the nature of the project. Participation was voluntary and anonymous, and it was stressed it did not imply any disadvantage for the student. Parents or caregivers gave passive written consent in accordance with the method suggested by Carroll-Lind, Chapman, Gregory, and Maxwell (2006), and adolescent participants gave verbal assent. Two researchers trained in collecting data on child victimization (UNICEF, 2012) administered the questionnaires in a class session in early 2012. Fewer than 3% of the sample chose not to participate. This multicenter study was conducted in accordance with the basic ethical principles of the Declaration of Helsinki in Seoul (World Medical Association, 2008) and the Code of Ethics of the Catalan Psychological Association (COPC, 1989), and it was approved by the IRB of the study's home institution. No compensation was offered to participants.

Measures

Sociodemographic data sheet

Sociodemographic information on adolescents and their parents' background (age, gender, country of birth, educational level, and occupation) was gathered using a data sheet created for the study.

Victimization experiences – juvenile victimization questionnaire

JVQ (Finkelhor et al., 2005) is a widely used self-report instrument designed to assess 34 different types of victimization against children and adolescents. The current JVQ version was previously translated into Catalan and Spanish. Two items regarding electronic victimization were added with the authors' permission in 2009, and later included in the revised version of the JVQ. The instrument collects information about multiple types of victimizations, including six modules: conventional crime (nine items), caregiver victimization (four items), victimization by peers and siblings (six items), sexual victimization (six items), witnessing and indirect victimization (nine items), and electronic victimization (two items). For each item, the presence or absence of the victimization experience was scored as 1 or 0 respectively. The original version of this instrument has shown good psychometric properties (Finkelhor et al., 2005), and its Spanish/Catalan adaptation also presents adequate validity (Pereda, Gallardo-Pujol, & Guilera, 2016).

Data analysis

First, we computed the total number of victimizations (out of 36 items) for each participant in the lifetime and past-year timeframe (Finkelhor et al., 2005). Then, we identified poly-victim groups for both timeframes by using the two different approaches reported in the scientific literature: (a) method 1: the one-above-the-mean number of different types of victimization experienced in the victim group as a whole; (b) method 2: based on the 10% of the sample who experienced the highest number of victimizations; and (c) method 3: using LCA, the clustering analysis recommended when the sample size is large. The R package poLCA (Linzer & Lewis, 2011) was used in the LCA. The appropriate number of classes and relative model fit was determined using the Bayesian information criterion (BIC) and the Akaike information criterion (AIC). The lowest BIC and AIC values indicate the optimal number of classes and better fit. As different initial parameter values may lead to different local maxima of the log-likelihood function, the model was run several times using the class-conditional response probabilities as the initial values for the estimation algorithm. SPSS v.21 was used for the remaining data analyses, with the level of statistical significance being set at $p < .05$.

Once the groups were obtained, the chi-square test (χ^2) was used to compare victims and poly-victims within each method in terms of lifetime and past-year rates of victimization modules, and then odds ratios (OR) were calculated to obtain the strength of association. The OR was considered statistically significant when its 95% confidence interval (CI) did not include the value 1, and was interpreted as follows: values above 1 indicated a higher prevalence of the specific victimization module among poly-victims, while values below 1 indicated a higher prevalence among victims. In addition, the Mann Whitney U test was used to compare victims and poly-victims for each method in terms of the mean number of lifetime and past-year victimizations.

In order to describe differences between youth who are identified by the analytical methods and those who are not, three groups of lifetime poly-victims were created: (a) poly-victims identified only by the top 10% approach, $n = 89$; (b) poly-victims identified solely by the LCA, excluding those poly-victims selected for the top 10% method, $n = 113$; and (c) poly-victims identified solely by the one-above-the-mean method excluding the top 10% and LCA, $n = 100$. The chi-square test (χ^2), the Fisher's exact test and the Kruskal-Wallis test were performed to compare sociodemographic variables among these groups. Analyses were also run for the past-year poly-victimization.

Finally, Cohen's κ was used to test the degree of agreement between pairs of methods. The mean value of agreement from all the pairs was obtained based on Hallgren (2012). Values were interpreted according to Viera and Garrett (2005) criteria.

Results

Descriptive analysis and group composition for each lifetime and past-year poly-victimization approach

Nine hundred and sixteen participants had experienced at least one type of victimization in their lifetime; thus 83% were lifetime victims. Seven hundred and fifty-seven adolescents (68.6%) reported at least one victimization experience during the past year and were classified as past-year victims.

Based on these groups, poly-victims were identified using three different methods (see lifetime poly-victims, Figure 1, and past-year poly-victims, Figure 2). The first method defined poly-victims as those who had suffered one above the mean number of types of victimization experienced by the victim group during their lifetime ($M = 3.85$, $SD = 2.73$) and the past year ($M = 2.86$, $SD = 2.19$). With this method, five and four types of victimization were the thresholds applied respectively. Two hundred and ninety-eight adolescents (27.0%) were defined as lifetime poly-victims; while 212 (19.2%) were considered past-year poly-

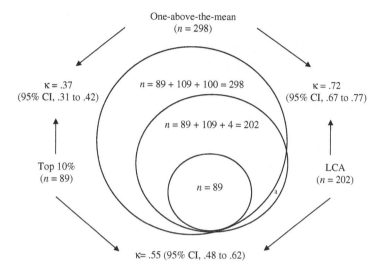

Figure 1. Degree of agreement between each pair of methods to assess lifetime poly-victimization. *Note.* [a]There are four poly-victim cases identified by LCA which are not selected with the other two methods.

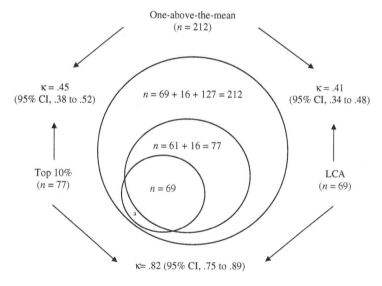

Figure 2. Degree of agreement between each pair of methods to assess past-year poly-victimization. *Note.* [a]There are eight poly-victim cases identified by LCA that are not selected with the other two methods.

victims. The second method was based on the 10% of the sample who experienced the highest number of victimizations. Cut-off points of eight and six types of victimization for lifetime and the past year, respectively, were used. Thus, 89 (8.1%) of the adolescents were identified as lifetime poly-victims, and 77 (7%) as past-year poly-victims. As regards the third approach, the LCA identified two classes in both timeframes; 69 (6.2%) adolescents were identified as poly-victims, who experienced a mean number of 7.83 (SD = 2.43) past-year victimizations, and 202 (18.3%) of them were identified as lifetime poly-victims with a mean number of 7.85 lifetime victimizations (SD = 2.42).

In all three methodologies, both lifetime and past-year poly-victims reported higher prevalences of each type of victimization than victims (see Tables 1 and 2), mainly conventional crimes, peer and sibling victimization, and witnessing and indirect victimization. Also, poly-victims were more likely to experience each type of victimization than victims. In this regard, in all lifetime methods the highest OR belonged to sexual victimization (ranging from 11.34 to 19.23) and conventional crimes (44.47), and the lowest to caregiver victimization (ranging from 4.28 to 4.29) and witnessing and indirect victimization (6.05). Moreover, regarding the past year, the three methods showed the highest OR for peer and sibling victimization (ranging from 11.51 to 23.78) and caregiver victimization (19.05), and the lowest for electronic victimization (ranging from 4.84 to 10.03) and witnessing and indirect victimization (4.24).

Regarding the number of victimization experiences during lifetime and the past year, poly-victims presented significantly more forms of victimization than victims (see last raw in Tables 1 and 2).

Comparison between poly-victims identified by each method

Regarding the type of poly-victims identified by each method, Table 3 shows the main sociodemographic characteristics for each group of lifetime poly-victims. Poly-victims identified solely by each method were comparable in terms of sex, country of birth, socioeconomic status, and age. Results for the past year are not reported because they are similar to the ones reported for the lifetime timeframe; they are available upon request from the authors.

Degree of agreement among the different methods to define poly-victimization

Regarding the lifetime, there was a fair agreement (κ = .37) between the one-above-the-mean number of victimizations and the top 10% approaches (see Figure 1). The LCA and the top 10% approaches showed moderate agreement (κ = .55), and the one-above-the-mean and the LCA approaches substantial agreement (κ = .72). The degree of agreement between methods was computed by an average of Cohen's κ across all rater pairs, obtaining moderate agreement: κ = .54 (95% CI, .49–.61).

Table 1. Descriptive statistics (%, M, SD, median, and OR) for JVQ victimization modules were shown for each lifetime poly-victimization approach.

Victimization modules	One-above-the-mean number of victimizations			Top 10%			LCA		
	Victims (n = 618)	Poly-victims (n = 298)	Statistic	Victims (n = 827)	Poly-victims (n = 89)	Statistic	Victims (n = 714)	Poly-victims (n = 202)	Statistic
	%	%	OR	%	%	OR	%	%	OR
Conventional crime	64.7	93.6	8.00***	71.3	100.0	1.15***	68.8	93.1	6.10***
Caregiver victimization	16.0	60.4	8.00***	25.4	77.5	10.14***	16.7	79.2	19.05***
Peer and sibling victimization	43.7	89.9	11.51***	54.7	96.6	23.78***	49.7	90.6	9.74***
Sexual victimization	4.0	24.2	7.56***	6.9	44.9	11.03***	4.2	33.2	11.32***
Witnessing and indirect victimization	47.1	82.9	5.44***	54.9	94.4	13.80***	52.1	82.2	4.24***
Electronic victimization	8.1	29.9	4.84***	10.9	55.1	10.03***	9.5	35.1	5.15***
	M (SD) Md	M (SD) Md		M (SD) Md	M (SD) Md		M (SD) Md	M (SD) Md	
Number of victimizations	2.32 (1.10) 2.00	7.05 (2.32) 6.00	0.00*** U^a	3.20 (1.84) 3.00	9.96 (2.11) 9.00	0.00*** U^a	2.72 (1.46) 2.00	7.85 (2.42) 7.00	2532.500*** U^a

Note. [a]Significance was shown by multiple asterisks. *p < .05, **p < .01, ***p < .001.

Table 2. Descriptive statistics (%, M, SD, median, and OR) for JVQ victimization modules were shown for each past-year poly-victimization approach.

	One-above-the-mean number of victimizations			Top 10%			LCA		
	Victims (n = 545)	Poly-victims (n = 212)	Statistic	Victims (n = 680)	Poly-victims (n = 77)	Statistic	Victims (n = 688)	Poly-victims (n = 69)	Statistic
Victimization modules	%	%	OR	%	%	OR	%	%	OR
Conventional crime	57.4	90.6	7.12***	63.1	98.7	44.47***	63.8	95.7	12.48***
Caregiver victimization	17.8	48.1	4.28***	22.6	58.4	4.80***	23.3	56.5	4.29***
Peer and sibling victimization	32.1	76.9	7.03***	39.6	89.6	13.18***	40.0	91.3	15.77***
Sexual victimization	2.4	21.7	11.34***	4.7	35.1	10.94***	4.1	44.9	19.23***
Witnessing and indirect victimization	35.8	74.5	5.25***	42.6	81.8	6.05***	43.5	78.3	4.68***
Electronic victimization	7.0	28.3	5.27***	9.9	40.3	6.17***	10.0	42.0	6.50***
	M (SD) Md	M (SD) Md	U^a	M (SD) Md	M (SD) Md	U^a	M (SD) Md	M (SD) Md	U^a
Number of victimizations	1.77 (.78) 2.00	5.64 (2.14) 5.00	.00***	2.30(1.29)2.00	7.78(2.24)7.00	.00***	2.36 (1.38) 2.00	7.83 (2.43) 7.00	522.50***

Note. ^aSignificance was shown by multiple asterisks. *p < .05, **p < .01, ***p < .001.

Table 3. Comparison of sociodemographic characteristics between lifetime poly-victim groups solely identified by each analytical method.

Sociodemographic variables	Only top 10% (n = 89)	Only LCA excluding top 10% (n = 113)	Only one-above-the-mean number of victimizations excluding top 10% and LCA (n = 100)	Statistic
	%	%	%	
Sex				$\chi^2_{(2)} = 4.782$
Male	52.8	46.0	61.0	
Female	47.2	54.0	39.0	
Country of origin				Fisher's exact test = 1.479
Spain	93.3	94.7	97.0	
Other	6.7	5.3	3.0	
SES[a]				$\chi^2_{(8)} = 6.070$
Low	1.2	3.9	0.0	
Middle low	8.2	9.8	8.4	
Middle	20.0	14.7	15.8	
Middle high	36.5	33.3	37.9	
High	34.1	38.2	37.9	
	M (SD)	M (SD)	M (SD)	Kruskal Wallis H test
Age	15.17 (1.44)	14.69 (1.73)	14.76 (1.73)	$H_{(2)} = 3.893$

Note.
[a]The SES comparison between poly-victim groups excluded the missing cases (only top 10%, n = 4; only LCA excluding top 10%, n = 11; and only one-above-the-mean number of victimizations excluding top 10% and LCA, n = 5).

Moreover, considering past-year, there was a moderate agreement ($\kappa = .41$) between the one-above-the-mean number of victimizations and the LCA approaches and also the top 10% and the one-above-the-mean approaches ($\kappa = .45$) (see Figure 2). Moreover, the top 10% and the LCA approaches showed an almost perfect agreement ($\kappa = .82$. Finally, the degree of agreement between methods was again computed by an average of Cohen's κ across all rater pairs, obtaining moderate agreement: $\kappa = .56$) (95% CI, .49–.63).

Discussion

The present study has focused on the comparison of the three different methodologies that previous studies have used to identify poly-victims using the JVQ (i.e., the one-above-the-mean number of victimizations, the top 10%, and LCA). The findings underline the need for a solid and reliable method to detect these children and youth in order to be able to offer them the resources they need.

Poly-victims are more likely to experience all forms of interpersonal violence than victims, no matter the method used to define the phenomenon. This shows, once again, the close relationship between the different forms of child victimization (Hamby & Grych, 2013), and should alert researchers to the need to use instruments that allow the assessment of a comprehensive list of violence experiences in childhood.

Poly-victims present differences with regard to the timeframe. Over the lifetime they mainly experience sexual victimization and conventional crimes, while over the past year they tend to experience more peer and sibling victimization and caregiver victimization.

Finkelhor et al. (2009) highlighted the specific influence of sexual and caregiver victimization in poly-victimization and recommended that these experiences should be weighted when using the JVQ, in view of the possibility that they might be reported with a higher frequency or chronicity and might have an important influence on the explanation of traumatic distress or on its intensity. The severity of both these experiences in child development has been confirmed in previous studies (Kendall-Tackett, 2003). Our results also show that children who suffered sexual or caregiver victimization are more prone to experiencing other victimization experiences and may have an increased risk of lifetime revictimization, as prospective studies have demonstrated (Widom, Czaja, & Dutton, 2008).

In addition, the fact that most poly-victims present a higher percentage of conventional crimes, and witnessing and indirect victimization outside the family, may be related to the frequent low self-control and risky lifestyles of adolescents (Cuevas, Finkelhor, Turner, & Ormord, 2007; Turanovic & Pratt, 2014; Vézina et al., 2011). Previous studies have found that exposure to groups, areas, and contexts with high levels of violence is similar in both victimization and offending processes (Fagan & Mazerolle, 2011; Jennings, Higgins, Tewksbury, Gover, & Piquero, 2010). Therefore, according to lifestyle and routine activity perspectives (Meier & Miethe, 1993), risky behaviors in adolescence increase the likelihood of extrafamilial victimization (Burrow & Apel, 2008; Schreck, Stewart, & Osgood, 2008; Smith & Ecob, 2007). Indeed, the frequent conjunction of witnessing intrafamilial violence and child abuse has also been demonstrated (Hamby, Finkelhor, Turner, & Ormrod, 2010), as well as connections between exposure to domestic violence and extrafamily victimization (Baldry, 2003).

Regarding the degree of agreement between the poly-victimization approaches, the results showed a moderate degree of consistency between the three methods used. Over the lifetime, the highest agreement was observed between the one-above-the-mean and LCA methods, whereas for identifying past-year poly-victims the highest degree of consistency was found between the top 10% and LCA methods. This suggests that they detect a similar group of adolescents. The lowest agreement obtained was between the two methods proposed by Finkelhor and colleagues (Finkelhor, Ormrod et al., 2005; Finkelhor et al., 2009) for the lifetime, and between LCA and the one-above-the-mean number of different victimization experiences during the last year.

The fact that LCA identify poly-victims by grouping their victimization profiles, while the other two methods select them by focusing on the number of victimizations, led us to hypothesize that the agreement between these approaches would be low. Overall however, taking both timeframes into account, we see that it is also quite rare to find agreement between methods based on the same approach. A possible explanation for the presence of a certain degree of disagreement between the methods may be the fact that the three methods solely identify different types of poly-victims in terms of their sociodemographic characteristics. However, results revealed that poly-victims identified or not identified by each method were comparable in terms of sex, country of birth, socioeconomic status, and age. It would be interesting to examine which poly-victims are or are not identified by each method with respect to the victimization events experienced. As seen in this paper, the relevance of the LCA method might suggest that identifying distinct profiles of poly-victimization empirically is important in addition to identifying individuals who have experienced a variety of combinations of multiple types of victimization.

Therefore, after this first research approximation, it is clear that poly-victimization researchers should continue to take into account the whole spectrum of multiple victimization experiences among children and youth. It is also clear that further research is needed to identify the best method for clinicians and researchers to use in order to select the children and adolescents most at risk of victimization.

Limitations

The study presents certain limitations that should be mentioned. The fact that the sample is not nationally representative should be kept in mind when interpreting the results obtained, as should the retrospective nature of the study. The lack of representativeness may explain the range and distribution of the number of victimizations observed, which in turn may determine the cut-off point obtained with the one-above-the-mean number of victimizations and the top 10% approaches. It should also be borne in mind that several versions of the JVQ are available with varying numbers of items (e.g., 36 in the adaptation by Pereda et al., 2014; and 34 in the adaptation by Cyr et al., 2013). The differences in the numbers of items and in the ways of counting the victimization experiences (i.e., Separate Item, Screener Sum, Separate Incident and Reduced Item Versions, see Finkelhor et al., 2005) may have a decisive influence on the results obtained.

Research needs and further questions

The use of different methods to define poly-victimization may result in the identification of different groups of poly-victims. This situation has serious implications for research and clinical practice. From a research perspective, the fact that some authors identify different kinds and different numbers of victims as poly-victims may lead to variations in the outcomes obtained related to this phenomenon. As for the clinical implications, even when the agreement between methods seems to be high, some children and adolescents may be left out of the poly-victim group and may thus be deprived of much-needed intervention. This is a particularly serious problem given the high number of violent situations they may experience (Cyr, Clément, & Chamberland, 2013). Also, experiencing at least one type of victimization makes youths more vulnerable to future victimization (Widom et al., 2008) and to the development of mental health problems (Turner et al., 2010).

There is no question that major progress has been made in developmental victimology. Perhaps it is now time to reflect upon certain questions in order to guide future advances in the field. First, when assessing the multiple experiences a child has suffered, researchers and practitioners should bear in mind that poly-victimization is a complex phenomenon that requires further analysis. They should also be aware that the use of a particular method to identify a group of poly-victims may fail to detect certain seriously victimized children. In consequence, issues, such as defining the most adequate approach or/and method to identify poly-victims or establishing the impact of using different forms of the same questionnaire (or even different questionnaires) to assess victimization should be carefully discussed. Secondly, when agreement has been reached regarding the operational definition of poly-victimization, future long-itudinal studies should explore whether the power of these approaches for predicting the consequences in later life remains similar over time.

Conclusions

This article describes a preliminary approach to the complex study of poly-victimization, for both lifetime and past-year time periods. Our results high-light the need for a method to identify poly-victims that makes it clear that we are talking about the same victims. The use of the same method for assessing poly-victimization will also allow comparisons between groups from different studies and above all to ensure that no poly-victims in need of treatment are neglected.

Funding

This research was funded and supported by research grants from Segimon Serrallonga scholarship, and the Spain's Ministerio de Economía y Competitividad (MEC) [grant number DER2012-38559-C03-02]. The authors declare no conflicts of interest.

References

Álvarez-Lister, M. S., Pereda, N., Abad, J., & Guilera, G.; The GReVIA. (2014). Polyvictimization and its relationship to symptoms of psychopathology in a southern European sample of adolescent outpatients. *Child Abuse & Neglect*, *38*(4), 747–756.

Baldry, A. C. (2003). Bullying in schools and exposure to domestic violence. *Child Abuse & Neglect*, *27*, 713–732. doi:10.1016/S0145-2134(03)00114-5

Bernstein, D. P., Ahluvalia, T., Pogge, D., & Handelsman, L. (1997). Validity of the childhood trauma questionnaire in an adolescent psychiatric population. *Journal of the American Academy of Child & Adolescent Psychiatry*, *36*, 340–348. doi:10.1097/00004583-199703000-00012

Burrow, J., & Apel, R. (2008). Youth behavior, school structure, and student risk of victimization. *Justice Quarterly*, *25*(2), 349–380. doi:10.1080/07418820802025181

Carroll-Lind, J., Chapman, J. W., Gregory, J., & Maxwell, G. (2006). The key to the gate keepers: Passive consent to and other ethical issues surrounding the rights of children to speak on issues that concern them. *Child Abuse & Neglect*, *30*(9), 979–989. doi:10.1016/j.chiabu.2005.11.013

Chan, K. L. (2013). Victimization and poly-victimization among school-aged Chinese adolescents: Prevalence and associations with health. *Preventive Medicine*, *56*(3–4), 207–210. doi:10.1016/j.ypmed.2012.12.018

Col·legi Oficial de Psicòlegs de Catalunya, COPC. (1989). *(Code of ethics) Codi deontològic.* Barcelona, Spain: Author.

Cook, A., Spinazzola, J., Ford, J., Lanktree, C., Blaustein, M., Cloitre, M, . . . Van Der Kolk, B. (2005). Complex trauma in children and adolescents. *Psychiatric Annals*, *35*, 390–398. doi:10.3928/00485713-20050501-05

Cuevas, C. A., Finkelhor, D., Turner, H. A., & Ormrod, R. K. (2007). Juvenile delinquency and victimization: A theoretical typology. *Journal of Interpersonal Violence*, *22*, 1581–1602. doi:10.1177/0886260507306498

Cyr, K., Chamberland, C., Clément, M. E., Lessard, G., Wemmers, J. A., Collin-Vézina, D., . . . Damant, D. (2013). Polyvictimization and victimization of children and youth: Results from a populational survey. *Child Abuse & Neglect*, *37*(10), 814–820. doi:10.1016/j.chiabu.2013.03.009

Cyr, K., Chamberland, C., Lessard, G., Clément, M.-È., Wemmers, J.-A., Collin-Vézina, D., . . . Damant, D. (2012). Polyvictimization in a child welfare sample of children and youths. *Psychology of Violence*, *2*(4), 385–400. doi:10.1037/a0028040

Cyr, K., Clément, M. E., & Chamberland, C. (2013). Lifetime prevalence of multiple victimizations and its impact on children's mental health. *Journal of Interpersonal Violence*, *29*(4), 616–634. doi:10.1177/0886260513505220

Dong, F., Cao, F., Cheng, P., Cui, N., & Li, Y. (2013). Prevalence and associated factors of poly-victimization in Chinese adolescents. *Scandinavian Journal of Psychology*, *54*, 415–422. doi:10.1111/sjop.12059

Fagan, A. A., & Mazerolle, P. (2011). Repeat offending and repeat victimization: Assessing similarities and differences in psychosocial risk factors. *Crime & Delinquency*, *57*, 732–755. doi:10.1177/0011128708321322

Finkelhor, D., Hamby, S. L., Ormrod, R., & Turner, H. (2005). The juvenile victimization questionnaire: Reliability, validity and national norms. *Child Abuse & Neglect, 29*(4), 383–412. doi:10.1016/j.chiabu.2004.11.001

Finkelhor, D., Ormrod, R., & Turner, H. (2009). Lifetime assessment of poly-victimization in a national sample of children and youth. *Child Abuse & Neglect, 33*(7), 403–411. doi:10.1016/j.chiabu.2008.09.012

Finkelhor, D., Ormrod, R., Turner, H., & Hamby, S. L. (2005). Measuring poly-victimization using the juvenile victimization questionnaire. *Child Abuse & Neglect, 29*(11), 1297–1312. doi:10.1016/j.chiabu.2005.06.005

Finkelhor, D., Ormrod, R. K., & Turner, H. A. (2007). Poly-victimization: A neglected component in child victimization. *Child Abuse & Neglect, 31*, 7–26. doi:10.1016/j.chiabu.2006.06.008

Ford, J. D., Grasso, D. J., Hawke, J., & Chapman, J. F. (2013). Poly-victimization among juvenile justice-involved youths. *Child Abuse & Neglect, 37*, 788–800. doi:10.1016/j.chiabu.2013.01.005

Gustafsson, P. E., Nilsson, D., & Svedin, C. G. (2009). Polytraumatization and psychological symptoms in children and adolescents. *European Child & Adolescent Psychiatry, 18*, 274–283. doi:10.1007/s00787-008-0728-2

Hallgren, K. A. (2012). Computing inter-rater reliability for observational data: An overview and tutorial. *Tutorials in Quantitative Methods for Psychology, 8*(1), 23–34. doi:10.20982/tqmp.08.1.p023

Hamby, S. L., & Finkelhor, D. (2000). The victimization of children: Recommendations for assessment and instrument development. *Journal of the American Academy of Child and Adolescent Psychiatry, 39*(7), 829–840. doi:10.1097/00004583-200007000-00011

Hamby, S., Finkelhor, D., Turner, H., & Ormrod, R. (2010). The overlap of witnessing partner violence with child maltreatment and other victimizations in a nationally representative survey of youth. *Child Abuse & Neglect, 34*(10), 734–741. doi:10.1016/j.chiabu.2010.03.001

Hamby, S. L., & Grych, J. (2013). *The web of violence: Exploring connections among different forms of interpersonal violence and abuse.* New York, NY: Springer. doi:10.1007/978-94-007-5596-3

Higgins, D. L., & McCabe, M. P. (2000). Multi-type maltreatment and the long-term adjustment of adults. *Child Abuse Review, 9*(1), 6–18. doi:10.1002/(SICI)1099-0852(200001/02)9:1<6::AID-CAR579>3.0.CO;2-W

Hollingshead, A. B. (1975). *Four factor index of social status.* Working paper. New Haven, CT: Yale University. Retrieved from http://www.yale.edu/sociology/yjs/yjs_fall_2011.pdf

Holt, M. K., Finkelhor, D., & Kaufman, G. (2007). Multiple experiences of urban elementary school students: Associations with psychological functioning and academic performance. *Child Abuse & Neglect, 31*, 503–515. doi:10.1016/j.chiabu.2006.12.006

Jennings, W. G., Higgins, G. E., Tewksbury, R., Gover, A. R., & Piquero, A. R. (2010). A longitudinal assessment of the victim-offender overlap. *Journal of Interpersonal Violence, 25*, 2147–2174. doi:10.1177/0886260509354888

Kendall-Tackett, K. A. (2003). *Treating the lifetime health effects of childhood victimization.* Kingston, NJ: Civic Research Institute, Inc.

Kretschmar, J. M., Tossone, K., Butcher, F., & Flannery, D. J. (2016). Patterns of poly-victimization in a sample of at-risk youth. *Journal of Child & Adolescent Trauma*, 1–13. doi:10.1007/s40653-016-0109-9

Le, M. T. H., Holton, S., Romero, L., & Fisher, J. (2016). Polyvictimization among children and adolescents in low- and lower-middle-income countries: A systematic review and meta-analysis. *Trauma, Violence, and Abuse.* doi:10.1177/1524838016659489

Linzer, D. A., & Lewis, J. B. (2011). poLCA: AN R package for polytomous variable latent class analysis. *Journal of Statistical Software, 42*(10), 1–29. doi:10.18637/jss.v042.i10

Meier, R. F., & Miethe, T. D. (1993). Understanding theories of criminal victimization. *Crime & Justice, 17,* 459–499. doi:10.1086/449218

Pereda, N., Gallardo-Pujol, D., & Guilera, G. (2016). Good practices in the assessment of victimization: The Spanish adaptation of the juvenile victimization questionnaire from a causal indicators approach. *Psychology of Violence.* doi:10.1037/vio0000075

Pereda, N., Guilera, G., & Abad, J. (2014). Victimization and polyvictimization of Spanish children and youth: Results from a community sample. *Child Abuse & Neglect, 38*(4), 640–649. doi:10.1016/j.chiabu.2014.01.019

Radford, L., Corral, S., Bradley, C., & Fisher, H. L. (2013). The prevalence and impact of child maltreatment and other types of victimization in the UK: Findings from a population survey of caregivers, children and young people and young adults. *Child Abuse & Neglect, 37*(10), 801–813. doi:10.1016/j.chiabu.2013.02.004

Reid, J. A., & Sullivan, C. J. (2009). A latent class typology of juvenile victims and exploration of risk factors and outcomes of victimization. *Criminal Justice and Behavior, 36,* 1001–1024. doi:10.1177/0093854809340621

Schreck, C. J., Stewart, E. A., & Osgood, D. W. (2008). A reappraisal of the overlap of violent offenders and victims. *Criminology; an Interdisciplinary Journal, 46*(4), 871–906. doi:10.1111/j.1745-9125.2008.00127.x

Smith, D. J., & Ecob, R. (2007). An investigation into causal links between victimization and offending in adolescents. *The British Journal of Sociology, 58*(4), 633–659. doi:10.1111/j.1468-4446.2007.00169.x

Sterzing, P. R., Ratliff, G. A., Gartner, R. E., McGeough, B. L., & Johnson, K. C. (2017). Social ecological correlates of polyvictimization among a national sample of transgender, genderqueer, and cisgender sexual minority adolescents. *Child Abuse & Neglect, 67,* 1–12. doi:10.1016/j.chiabu.2017.02.017

Turanovic, J. J., & Pratt, T. C. (2014). "Can't stop, won't stop": Self-Control, risky lifestyles, and repeat victimization. *Journal of Quantitative Criminology, 30*(1), 29–56. doi:10.1007/s10940-012-9188-4

Turner, H. A., Finkelhor, D., & Ormrod, R. (2006). The effect of lifetime victimization on the mental health of children and adolescents. *Social Science and Medicine, 62*(1), 13–27. doi:10.1016/j.socscimed.2005.05.030

Turner, H. A., Finkelhor, D., & Ormrod, R. (2010). Poly-victimization in a national sample of children and youth. *American Journal of Preventive Medicine, 38,* 323–330. doi:10.1016/j.amepre.2009.11.012

Turner, H. A., Shattuck, A., Finkelhor, D., & Hamby, S. (2016). Polyvictimization and youth violence exposure across contexts. *Journal of Adolescent Health, 58,* 208–214. doi:10.1016/j.jadohealth.2015.09.021

United Nations Children Fund (UNICEF). (2012). *Ethical principles, dilemmas and risks in collecting data on violence against children: A review of available literature.* New York, NY: UNICEF, Statistics and Monitoring Section, Division of Policy and Strategy. Retrieved from http://www.childinfo.org/files/Childprotection_EPDRCLitReview_final_lowres.pdf

Vézina, J., Hébert, M., Poulin, F., Lavoie, F., Vitaro, F., & Tremblay, R. E. (2011). Risky lifestyle as a mediator of the relationship between deviant peer affiliation and dating violence victimization among adolescent girls. *Journal of Youth and Adolescence, 40*(7), 814–824. doi:10.1007/s10964-010-9602-x

Viera, A. J., & Garrett, J. M. (2005). Understanding interobserver agreement: The Kappa statistic. *Family Medicine, 37*(5), 360–363. Retrieved from http://www.stfm.org/FamilyMedicine/Vol37Issue5/Viera360

Walsh, C. A., MacMillan, H. L., Trocmé, N., Jamieson, E., & Boyle, M. H. (2008). Measurement of victimization in adolescence: Development and validation of the child-hood experiences of violence questionnaire. *Child Abuse & Neglect, 32,* 1037–1057. doi:10.1016/j.chiabu.2008.05.003

Widom, C. S., Czaja, S. J., & Dutton, M. A. (2008). Childhood victimization and lifetime revictimization. *Child Abuse & Neglect, 32*(8), 785–796. doi:10.1016/j.chiabu.2007.12.006

Widom, C. S., Raphael, K. G., & DuMont, K. A. (2004). The case for prospective longitudinal studies in child maltreatment research: Commentary on Dube, Williamson, Thompson, Felitti, and Anda (2004). *Child Abuse & Neglect, 28*(7), 715–722. doi:10.1016/j.chiabu.2004.03.009

World Medical Association. (2008). *WMA declaration of helsinki. Ethical principles for medical research involving human subjects.* Seoul, Republic of Korea: 59th WMA General Assembly. Retrieved from http://www.wma.net/en/30publications/10policies/b3/

Zolotor, A. J., Runyan, D. K., Dunne, M. P., Jain, D., Ramirez, C., Volkova, C., ... Isaeva, O. (2009). ISPCAN child abuse screening tool children's version (ICAST-C): Instrument development and multi-national pilot testing. *Child Abuse & Neglect, 33,* 833–841. doi:10.1016/j.chiabu.2009.09.004

2 Polyvictimization and externalizing symptoms in foster care children

The moderating role of executive function

Sarah R. Horn, Leslie E. Roos, Kathryn G. Beauchamp, Jessica E. Flannery, and Philip A. Fisher

ABSTRACT

Prior research has identified the role of childhood maltreatment in externalizing problems and executive function (EF) deficits, but minimal work has been done to characterize the effects of co-occurring maltreatment types, defined as polyvictimization. Here, we sought to characterize the association between polyvictimization and externalizing problems in a sample of foster care children aged 3–4 years ($N = 84$) and examine how EF may mediate or moderate that relationship. A moderation model was supported in that only polyvictimized children with EF scores 1.62 or more standard deviations below the mean were at heightened risk for clinically severe externalizing problems, while no association between polyvictimization and externalizing problems were observed for children who scored at the mean or above on the EF measure. Findings highlight that EF may serve as a resilience factor indicating that individual differences in polyvictimized children's EF skills help to predict variability in externalizing problems. Future research on designing and optimizing intervention programs that target EF skills may mitigate the development of maladaptive outcomes for polyvictimized children.

Young children in foster care are disproportionately more likely to experience polyvictimization (i.e., multiple types of maltreatment; Pears, Kim, & Fisher, 2008) and, in turn, are at elevated risk for negative outcomes (Leeb, Lewis, & Zolotor, 2011). In a cross-sectional survey of children's exposure to violence, 49% of the children surveyed suffered two or more types of polyvictimization (Finkelhor et al., 2011); for children in foster care, rates of polyvictimization may be as high as 95% (Lau et al., 2005; Manly, Kim, Rogosch, & Cicchetti, 2001). Prior maltreatment research has largely focused on specific forms of abuse or neglect. In contrast, children's actual experiences often involve more than one type of maltreatment (Greeson et al., 2011; Turner, Finkelhor, & Ormrod, 2010). It is important to note that a wide range of variability exists not only in children's experiences of victimization types but *also* in the risk for associated negative outcomes.

A related issue among foster children is the documented presence of externalizing problems (e.g., defiance, aggression, impulsivity) commonly observed above and beyond other mental health issues (Stein, Mazumdar, & Rae-Grant, 1996). Of concern, externalizing symptoms are often precursors to negative outcomes, such as risk-taking, antisocial behavior, and suicidality (Campbell, Shaw, & Gilliom, 2000). Despite numerous studies documenting the high *prevalence* of externalizing problems in young children in foster care, ranging from 20% to 78% (Keil & Price, 2006), there is relatively little research investigating how variation in children's maltreatment experiences is associated with externalizing risk within foster care samples. Heterogeneity in individuals' responses to maltreatment is an important challenge for both researchers and practitioners (Afifi & MacMillan, 2011). Polyvictimization quantifies variability in maltreatment experiences to disentangle individual differences in externalizing problem risk. Focusing on the number of maltreatment types experienced is a promising approach to operationalizing polyvictimization (Cecil, Viding, Fearon, Glaser, & McCrory, 2017).

Polyvictimization and externalizing behavior

Externalizing problems are often observed in samples of polyvictimized children in foster care and community populations (Cyr et al., 2012; Turner et al., 2010). Theoretical perspectives lend insight into this association. From a social learning perspective, externalizing behavior can be conceptualized as modeling of observed parental behavior (Patterson & Yoerger, 2002). Per social learning theory, a child both witnessing domestic violence and experiencing physical abuse may have observed aggression and frequently engaged in coercive parenting interactions that urge the child to imitate the modeled behavior (Moylan et al., 2010). Experiences of multiple maltreatment types increase the repertoire of modeled behaviors from which children learn, thereby increasing the likelihood of similar violence perpetration. Attachment theory suggests that the lack of a responsive attachment figure within contexts of polyvictimization contributes to risk for externalizing behavior via the child's failure to develop effective self-regulatory emotional and behavioral strategies for dealing with distress, which is likely to be more pervasive across contexts in situations of polyvictimization (Stovall-McClough & Dozier, 2004). While supportive caregiving and authoritative discipline are associated with regulatory capacities (Kochanska, Murray, & Harlan, 2000; Spinrad et al., 2007), harsh discipline is linked to impaired self-regulatory capacities in children, including deficits in inhibitory control and behavioral regulation (Olson et al., 2011). In turn, diminished self-regulatory capacities may increase the risk for externalizing behavior (Fay-Stammbach, Hawes, & Meredith, 2014).

Numerous studies have demonstrated a robust link between early adversity and a range of externalizing behavior problems (e.g., aggression, delinquency). Several mediators and moderators underlying this relationship have been identified, such as emotion regulation (Kim & Cicchetti, 2010), parenting styles (Lansford et al., 2006), and compromised attention (Roman, Ensor, & Hughes, 2016). A study of community children aged 4–15 years found that externalizing problems significantly increased for each additional adverse event exposure (Fleckman, Drury, Taylor, & Theall, 2016). Few studies have investigated the risk of externalizing behavior in the context of polyvictimization; it is essential to further delineate the complex relationship between co-occurring victimizations and externalizing symptomatology.

Executive function as a mediator or moderator in the path from polyvicimtization to externalizing problems

Executive functions (EF), or the higher-order cognitive processes supporting goal-directed behavior, are considered a core capacity predictive of adaptive functioning (Garon, Bryson, & Smith, 2008). EF is considered to comprise at least three key subdomains—inhibitory control, working memory, and mental flexibility (Garon, Bryson, & Smith, 2008). Germane to the present investigation, deficits in EF appear to be strongly related to externalizing behavior in young maltreated children; a recent meta-analysis of primarily community-based studies reported a medium effect size for the association between EF and externalizing behavior (Schoemaker, Mulder, Deković, & Matthys, 2013). Attention is fundamentally involved in several EF component operations (Barkley, 1996) and the development of EF skills in preschool-aged children may be in large part due to the role of attention (Garon et al., 2008). Further, performance on EF tasks is highly correlated with attention processes (Kane & Engle, 2003; Miller & Marcovitch, 2015).

The extent to which EF may be a mediator or a moderator in the association between polyvictimization and externalizing problems is a critical open question. Most extant work on this topic has focused on EF's role in the association between parental risk and externalizing behavior, which may inform the development of conceptual models to describe how a range of early experiences impact EF and, in turn, externalizing behavior. Child EF at age 3 has been shown to mediate the relationship between maternal depressive symptoms and externalizing problems at age 6 years (Roman et al., 2016). In a sample of families living in rural poverty, EF mediated the association between sensitive parenting and lower externalizing behavior longitudinally across early childhood (Sulik, Blair, Mills-Koonce, Berry, &

Greenberg, 2015). These data suggest that EF skills may explain the link between maltreatment and externalizing behavior.

Evidence also exists for EF as a moderator, such that children with high EF demonstrate resilience following maltreatment, including lower risk for externalizing behavior, compared to children with low EF (Obradović, 2010). Attention skills have also been shown to moderate the link between maltreatment intensity and academic performance (Slade & Wissow, 2007). Such findings provide support for a resilience factor model, in which certain factors can either buffer children or heighten the risks of the negative impacts of early life adversity (Masten, 2001). EF skills are hypothesized to serve as a protective *or* risk factor underlying the link between polyvictimization and externalizing behaviors, in that deficits in EF place young children at particularly high risk for maladaptive outcomes while above average EF skills may buffer against the negative impacts of early life adversity.

Current study

Given the limited previous research examining links between polyvictimization and externalizing symptoms within maltreated samples, we first sought to examine the extent to which polyvictimization increased risk for externalizing problems (defined as those in the borderline, or clinical range) in a secondary data analysis from a sample of foster care children. Polyvictimization was operationalized as the number of different maltreatment types experienced. We hypothesized that children with higher polyvictimization would be at elevated risk for externalizing problems. Next, we tested the relationship between polyvictimization and externalizing behaviors and investigated the role of EF in mediation and moderation models. Given support for both models in the literature, and a dearth of studies in polyvictimized samples, we did not have a specific hypothesis regarding whether EF would mediate or moderate the association between polyvictimization and externalizing problems. A mediation model would suggest that EF accounts for the link between polyvictimization and externalizing behaviors while a moderation model would indicate individual differences in children's EF skills place them at variable risk for externalizing problems, given a history of polyvictimization (see Figure 1).

Method

Participants

The sample comprised a subgroup of participants from a randomized controlled trial (RCT) of Multidimensional Foster Care for Preschoolers (MTFC-P; Fisher, Gunnar, Chamberlain, & Reid, 2000), which included children

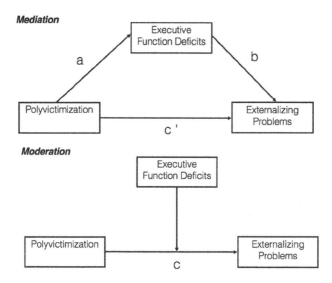

Figure 1. Hypothesized mediation and moderation models.

aged 3–6 years who were entering a new foster care placement between 2000 and 2003. The original sample included 117 maltreated foster care children (63 males) recruited from a mid-sized urban area in the Pacific Northwest participating in the RCT. For this study, we combined foster treatment and foster comparison arms into a single group for analysis. An additional 60 children were recruited from the community as a comparison sample. The community sample was recruited from the same geographic area and from low income households. The "community controls" had no history of child welfare involvement. While community controls are not the focus of the present study as they had no polyvictimization data, they are briefly included throughout the methods and measures to demonstrate the extent to which children in foster care exhibited functional impairment compared to community controls.

The present study analyzed foster care and community children aged 3–4 years due to an age restriction on the EF measure. Therefore, the sample was reduced to $N = 88$ foster care children and $N = 47$ community controls. For analyses comparing foster care children to the community controls on externalizing problems and EF scores, the full subsample was utilized. However, for analyses examining polyvictimization, EF, and externalizing problems, we only used the foster care sample.

Sociodemographic variables

The ethnicity of the sample reflects the local community: In the foster care sample, the ethnicity breakdown was: 88.9% Caucasian, 4.3% Native

American, 5.1% mixed race/other, .9% Latino, and .9% African-American. In the community sample, 76.7% of the children were Caucasian, 6.7% Native-American, 6.7% mixed race/other, 1.7% Latino, and 6.7% African-American. In the foster care sample, 53.8% ($n = 63$) of the children were male and the average age was 4.04 years ($SD = .85$). In the community sample, the average age was 4.33 ($SD = 0.79$) and 53.5% of the sample was male ($n = 32$).

Measures

Study measures were collected from children and foster parents in laboratory and home-based assessments after obtaining informed consent to participate in the research study. All procedures were developed in partnership with the local and state child welfare agencies and were approved by the Institutional Review Board.

Maltreatment profiles

The Maltreatment Classification System (MCS; Barnett, Manly, & Cicchetti, 1993) was utilized to code child welfare system (CWS) case records for lifetime maltreatment histories. The MCS codes for several types of maltreatment, including: physical abuse, sexual abuse, failure to provide (e.g., parental failure to provide adequate food, clothing, or a safe living environment), supervisory neglect (e.g., parental failure to provide age-appropriate supervision), emotional maltreatment (e.g., parental rejection, allowing the child to witness traumatic events), educational maltreatment (i.e., parental failure to send the child to school), and moral/legal maltreatment (i.e., parents using the child for illegal purposes). The rates for the latter two categories were extremely low: educational maltreatment ($n = 9$) and moral/legal maltreatment ($n = 1$). Because of the low base rates and the distinct nature of these categories, these two maltreatment types were dropped from further score calculation and analyses. The most common types of maltreatment experienced for the children aged 3–4 years were emotional neglect (90.9%), supervisory neglect (88.6%), and physical neglect (79.5%). Roughly one quarter of the foster care sample experienced physical or sexual abuse (Table 1).

Coding process

Caseworkers and the local child welfare agency consented to the review of case records. A child welfare representative excluded identifiable information. Coders completed extensive training on confidentiality agreements. Narratives of CWS referrals contained material about the specific types of maltreatment reported and investigated; however, narratives did not necessarily contain information on each type of maltreatment coded per MCS. Coders identified distinct maltreatment incidents from the narratives. To

Table 1. Descriptive statistics for the maltreatment variables.

Maltreatment type	Number of children	Percent of incidence
Physical abuse	24	27.3
Sexual abuse	20	22.7
Physical neglect	70	79.5
Supervisory neglect	78	88.6
Emotional maltreatment	80	90.9
Polyvictimization rates		
One maltreatment type	4	4.5
Two maltreatment types	20	22.7
Three maltreatment types	34	38.6
Four maltreatment types	24	27.3
Five maltreatment types	6	6.8

qualify as an incident, the event had to fit the MCS definitions of maltreatment and had to be reported by a mandatory reporter or caseworker. Maltreatment incidents were coded per type using the MCS.

Case records were coded by two coders who had been trained by an MCS author (Manley). To compute interrater agreement, 20% of the case records were double-coded. Overall, agreement on identification of incidents was high (80%). The average kappa was .72 across all the categories (physical abuse $\kappa = .82$, sexual abuse $\kappa = .67$, failure to provide $\kappa = .65$, supervisory neglect $\kappa = .65$, emotional maltreatment $\kappa = .79$).

Polyvictimization

Polyvictimization was conceptualized as a continuous measure of number of types of maltreatment experienced. Subject maltreatment types were coded from 0 to 5, with 0 indicating no maltreatment up to the maximum of 5 discrete maltreatment types. Overall, polyvictimization was frequent, with children experiencing an average of three different types of maltreatment. To note, 95.5% of this sample experienced polyvictimization, which is comparable to other maltreated samples (Lau et al., 2005; Manly et al., 2001).

Executive functioning

NEPSY: a developmental neuropsychological assessment

Children completed the NEPSY (Korkman, Kemp, & Kirk, 1998), which includes a series of 36 subtests assessing neuropsychological development across five domains, from which we specifically examined the Attention/Executive Functioning domain (other domains: Language, Sensorimotor, Visuospatial, and Memory and Learning). The EF domain assesses children's inhibition, self-regulation, and selective and sustained attention through two subtests.

Visual attention subtest

This subtest assesses children's speed and accuracy by instructing children to maintain attention and focus selectively on a visual target within a display. The first task is a simple selective attention task. The child is instructed to quickly locate and mark a picture of a bunny from various pictures in a linear array. Additionally, the child must search for pictures of a cat embedded within a random array of varying pictures.

Statue subtest

The statue subtest is designed to assess motor persistence and inhibition. Children are instructed to maintain a body position with their eyes closed for a 75 second period and to restrain any impulse to respond to sound distracters. Sound distractors include a pencil dropping, coughing, knocking on the table twice, saying "ho hum" and "time's up." A low score is indicative of poor inhibitory control and motor persistence.

Children in the foster care sample had a significantly lower average EF NEPSY scores of 93.11 ($SD = 15.02$) compared to the community sample average score of 99.24 ($SD = 12.75$) ($t(128) = -2.34$, $p = 0.021$).

Externalizing problems

Child behavior checklist

The CBCL (Achenbach, 1991) is a 112-item caregiver report for identifying problem behaviors in children. Caregivers rated children's behavior over the preceding 2 months on a 3-point scale (not true, somewhat/sometimes true, and very true/often true). The items yield a total score and two composite scores – Internalizing and Externalizing. The Externalizing subscale includes symptoms related to hyperactivity, defiance, aggression, and noncompliance. The CBCL externalizing subscale was dichotomized using a cut-off of T-scores ≥ 60, following the recommended guidelines for referral to clinical services.

In the foster sample, 54.5% ($N = 48$) of the children met the cut-off indicating clinical levels of externalizing behavior symptomatology compared to 12.8% of the community sample ($N = 6$; $t(133) = 5.13$, $p < 0.001$).

Data analysis plan

We first assessed bivariate correlations between the variables of interest in the foster care children. This step included bivariate correlations with sociodemographic and CWS-related covariates to assess which covariates were related to EF and/or externalizing behaviors. All covariates significantly associated with either variable were included in subsequent moderation and mediation analyses. Next, we tested the relationship between polyvictimization and externalizing behaviors, investigating the role of EF in mediation

Table 2. Zero-order correlations among the variables.

	Variable	1	2	3	4	5	6	7	8
1	Age	-	.09	-.08	-.01	.09	.12	.16	.15
2	Gender	-	-	.05	.06	-.01	.07	.32*	.14
3	Maternal education	-	-	-	.14	-.13	.01	.03	.01
4	Household income	-	-	-	-	.13	.30	-.07	.09
5	Number of transitions	-	-	-	-	-	.09	-.18	.11
6	Externalizing Problems	-	-	-	-	-	-	-.13	.16
7	EF NEPSY Score	-	-	-	-	-	-	-	.09
8	Polyvictimization	-	-	-	-	-	-	-	-

*p < .001

and moderation models. Specifically, we investigated the extent to which EF served as a mediator of the hypothesized association between polyvictimization and externalizing problems. We further investigated EF as a moderator of the hypothesized association between polyvictimization and externalizing problems, testing if high EF would be a protective factor from the presence of externalizing behaviors given a polyvictimization history.

Results

Preliminary covariate analyses

Zero-order correlations between all variables of interest and potential confounders, including age, number of out-of-home placements, maternal education, and gross annual household income were conducted (Table 2). Gender differences were examined with an independent t-test. Lower gross annual household income was positively correlated with externalizing problems ($r = 0.31$, $p < .001$). Age, number of transitions, and maternal education were not significantly correlated with any variables of interest (p-values > .083). There was a significant effect of gender on EF performance with boys performing worse than girls ($t(128) = -3.78$, $p < .001$). Accordingly, gender and annual household income were considered as covariates in subsequent multivariate analyses.

Multivariate analyses

To test baseline EF as a potential mediator or moderator linking polyvictimization to elevated externalizing problems, the PROCESS add-on module of SPSS v.22 was utilized (Hayes, 2013).

Missing data

Four children did not have complete data on the EF domain and were dropped from multivariate analyses due to listwise deletion procedures. Children who were missing data on the NEPSY test were more likely to have primary caregivers with lower education ($t(134) = 59.03$, $p < 0.001$). For all multivariate analyses, a sample size of $N = 84$ was included.

Mediation analysis

Polyvictimization was not associated with externalizing problems in initial bivariate correlations ($R^2 = .16$, $p = .15$; Figure 1, Path-C). Further, there was no association between polyvictimization and EF ($R^2 = .09$, $p = .43$); Figure 1, Path-A) or EF and externalizing ($R^2 = -13$, $p = .14$; Figure 1, Path-B). The model predicting EF from polyvictimization, gender, and household income was significant ($F(3, 76) = 5.07$, $R^2 = .18$, $p = .003$). Male gender predicted externalizing ($\beta = 11.54$, $SE = 3.09$, $p < .001$); no other predictors were significant. The overall model predicting externalizing from polyvictimization, gender, income, and EF was not significant (Cox & Snell's $R^2 = .05$, $p = .35$). No relation was observed between externalizing problems and any other variables, although there was a trend level direct effect for polyvictimization on externalizing in the full model ($\beta = .43$, $SE = .26$, $p = .09$). No evidence was observed for an indirect effect of polyvictimization on externalizing problems through EF ($\beta = -.03$, bootstrap $SE = .07$, bootstrap CI = [−0.25 to −0.04], indicating no support for a mediation model.

Moderation analysis

A moderation analysis was conducted predicting externalizing problems from polyvictimization, EF, an interaction of polyvicimtization × EF, considering gender and household income covariates. In this model, polyvictimization was a trend level predictor of externalizing problems ($\beta = .49$, $SE = .28$, $p = .08$). The polyvicimtization × EF interaction was a significant predictor of externalizing problems ($\beta = -.05$, $SE = .02$, $p = .026$). Neither EF nor the covariates were significant predictors of externalizing problems. Although the full logistic model, with covariates, was close to significant (Cox & Snell's $R^2 = 0.12$, $p = .07$), results indicated that this overall model did not explain significant variance in externalizing problems. To improve data fit, we removed non-significant covariates (gender and income; $p > .38$), resulting in a significant model fit (Cox & Snell's $R^2 = .11$, $p = .02$) with a similar pattern observed across predictors. In this final model, there was a trend level effect of polyvictimization on externalizing problems ($\beta = .47$, $SE = .26$, $p = .08$) and the interaction of polyvicimtization × EF remained significant ($\beta = -.04$, $SE = .02$, $p = .04$). There was no significant direct effect of EF on externalizing problems ($\beta = -028$, $SE = .17$, $p = .10$).

Conditional effects probing the polyvicimtization × EF interaction from the final model are shown in Figure 2. The interaction was probed by testing the conditional effects of externalizing behavior at three levels of EF: one standard deviation (SD) below the mean (score = 78.09), at the mean ($M = 93.11$), and one SD above the mean (score = 108.13). As demonstrated

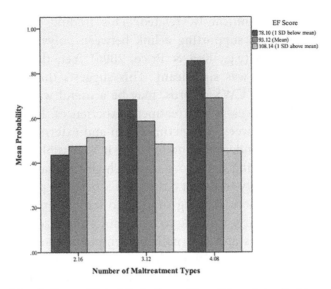

Figure 2. Conditional effects of Polyvictimization × EF on Externalizing Problems.

Table 3. Conditional effects of polyvictimization on externalizing problems at different levels of executive function.

Executive function value	β (SE) Polyvictimization on externalizing	p	95% CI
One SD below the mean (78.09)	1.061 (.423)	0.012	[0.236–2.001]
At the mean (M = 93.11)	0.468 (.265)	0.078	[−0.074–1.011]
One SD above the mean (108.13)	−0.125 (.367)	0.732	[−0.920–0.558]

in Table 3, externalizing problems were significantly related to polyvicimtization only when EF was below the mean ($\beta = 1.06$, SE $= 0.42$, $p = .01$), but not when EF was at or above the mean. The Johnson–Neyman technique demonstrated that the relationship between externalizing problems and polyvictimization was significant when EF scores fell 1.62 SD below the mean score of 93.11 (e.g., an EF score ≤ 91.49), but insignificant with EF scores higher than 91.49.

Discussion

Polyvictimization was highly prevalent in the present sample, as most of the children experienced three or more discrete types of maltreatment exposure, consistent with other high-risk samples (Lau et al., 2005; Manly et al., 2001). Externalizing problems were of clinical concern for the majority of this sample (57.3%), in line with prior research that maltreated children often exhibit elevated externalizing problems (Fleckman et al., 2016). Contrary to our first hypothesis, the final model indicated that polyvictimization and externalizing problems were marginally, but not significantly, related. This finding was unexpected, given the rich literature supporting a link between polyvictimization and externalizing behaviors (e.g., Keil & Price, 2006). Yet, the interaction of polyvictimization × EF was significant. This suggests that polyvictimization, as quantified from CWS records, may be a useful way of parameterizing individual differences in maltreatment experiences. Findings indicate that the relationship between polyvictimization and externalizing problems may be contingent on underlying moderators. It is possible, given the high prevalence of externalizing behaviors in this high-risk sample, that there was insufficient variability to detect a direct link between polyvictimization and externalizing behaviors, lending support to the notion that underlying moderators are particularly valuable to delineating the association between early adverse experiences and externalizing symptomatology.

Results extend prior work which has linked maltreatment experiences with risk for the development of externalizing behavior following single victimization exposure, such as physical abuse (Lansford et al., 2002) or childhood sexual abuse (Jones et al., 2013). While informative, given the high rates of polyvicimtization within maltreated populations, it is difficult and potentially of limited clinical utility to characterize the impact of a specific maltreatment type in isolation. The current study sought to address this gap by examining the role of polyvictimization in predicting externalizing symptomatology. We endeavored to build upon the knowledge base in this area by considering the role of EF skills – deficits documented in children with externalizing behaviors (Schoemaker et al., 2013).

EF is a key mechanism of interest in maltreated youth populations as prior research has demonstrated that children in high-risk samples often exhibit lower levels of EF (Roos, Kim, Schnabler, & Fisher, 2016). Consistently, foster children in this sample had significantly lower EF skills compared to the community controls. As noted, the literature has provided support for both mediation and moderation models of EF in the context of adversity in a variety of developmental stages (Obradović, 2010; Sulik et al., 2015).

The present study did not support a mediation model, suggesting that EF does not fully account for the link between polyvictimization and externalizing symptomatology in our sample. Rather, our results supported a moderation model, indicating that individual differences in polyvictimized children's EF skills serve as a factor in predicting externalizing problems and that only children with low EF scores were at high risk for externalizing problems following polyvictimization. Polyvictimized children with average, or above average, EF scores were buffered against externalizing problems. Findings are in line with previous research demonstrating that higher EF aptitude predicts resilient functioning following adversity; in a study of homeless youth, children's EF emerged as the strongest predictor of adaptive functioning, including lower levels of externalizing behaviors (Obradović, 2010). One possibility is that children with higher EF had more supportive parenting, even within the context of polyvictimization, contributing to enhanced EF and better behavior regulation (i.e., lower externalizing problems). Positive parenting practices are associated with both greater EF and regulatory capacities (Bernier, Carlson, & Whipple, 2010).

Inconsistent findings in the literature in characterizing EF as a mediator or moderator between maltreatment profiles and externalizing symptoms may be due in part to several factors, such as the limited number of studies, measures of EF utilized, the operationalization of maltreatment/polyvictimization, and the developmental age group investigated. Indubitably, EF plays a significant underlying role between maltreatment, polyvictimization, and externalizing symptoms and should continue to be explored in a myriad of samples.

Implications

Externalizing problems observed at young ages place children at higher risk for future maladaptive outcomes and trajectories, including risk-taking, substance abuse, and incarceration (Campbell et al., 2000), and polyvictimization is a key risk factor. Externalizing problems are among the most reported behavioral issues in early childhood (Keenan & Wakschlag, 2004), comprising up to one half of mental health service referrals (Belsky, Melhuish, Barnes, Leyland, & Romaniuk, 2006). Without intervention, externalizing problems often remain stable and may increase from preschool across the lifespan (Stormont, 2002). Therefore, identifying young children at the highest risk of developing externalizing problems may ameliorate the likelihood of maladaptive trajectories. Our study suggests that EF skills may be useful in identifying maltreated children at the highest risk for externalizing problems.

EF may help identify children at highest risk and inform intervention design and optimization, potentially decreasing the development or exacerbation of early externalizing problems. While the research on this topic is limited, preliminary studies are promising. One intervention designed to enhance school readiness in foster care children, Kids in Transition to School (KITS), demonstrated significant positive impacts on children's self-regulatory skills, key components related to EF (Pears et al., 2013). A separate program for socioeconomically disadvantaged children found that baseline EF skills in 4-year-old children moderated the impact of the intervention on several positive outcomes (Bierman, Nix, Greenberg, Blair, & Domitrovich, 2008). EF is also a malleable skill, potentially responsive to therapeutic techniques and interventions (Diamond & Lee, 2011).

Results support that EF can serve both as buffering *and* a risk factor following adversity. For example, children with low EF could be more likely than those with higher EF skills to model negative behaviors (e.g., social learning theory) or be more affected by the lack of sensitive and responsive caregiving (e.g., attachment theory), placing them at elevated risk for developing externalizing problems following polyvictimization.

Limitations

Given the nature of secondary data analysis, our study was limited to one measure of EF from a subdomain of an overall neuropsychological test and the subtests (e.g., Visual Attention) could not be computed. Future research would benefit from replicating findings using more standardized EF tasks, such as the Flanker task and dimensional change card sort (Gershon et al., 2013). However, the NEPSY and its subtests have been used as a measure of EF for preschool-aged children in other studies (e.g., Klenberg, Korkman, & Lahti-Nuuttila, 2001; Thorell & Wåhlstedt, 2006). In the MCS, reasons necessitating out-of-home care (e.g., domestic violence) are not part of the coding system and may have been coded under other types of maltreatment (e.g., emotional neglect), potentially inflating the prevalence. Further, missing data on the NEPSY reduced the sample size for the moderation model; results were not missing at random in that children whose mothers reported lower education were less likely to have participated in the EF test. Therefore, results may be less applicable for children with lower educated caregivers. Lastly, results may be less generalizable to more racially or ethnically diverse samples. Despite these limitations, the study was adequately powered to explore the moderating role of EF in the context of polyvictimization and externalizing problems.

Future directions

Future research can build upon such findings to explore the trajectories of children at highest risk due to lower EF skills, such as conducting longitudinal analyses to explore how baseline lower EF and attention skills predict children's well-being over time. Intervention programs that target EF skills may be critical for polyvictimized children and may mitigate the likelihood of developing externalizing problems, thus increasing the likelihood of healthier trajectories for these children across the lifespan.

Acknowledgments

Research support was provided by the following grants: R01 MH059780, NIMH, U.S. PHS; R21 MH065046; and R01 DA021424, NIDA, U.S. PHS.

Philip A. Fisher received support from NIH grants R01 HD075716 and P50 DA035763.
Leslie E. Roos received support from HHS-2014-ACF-ACYF-CA-0803.

References

Achenbach, T. M. (1991). *Child Behavior Checklist/4-18*. Burlington, VT: University of Vermont, Dept. of psychiatry.

Afifi, T. O., & MacMillan, H. L. (2011). Resilience following child maltreatment: A review of protective factors. *The Canadian Journal of Psychiatry*, *56*(5), 266–272. doi:10.1177/070674371105600505

Barkley, R. A. (1996). Linkages between attention and executive functions. In G. R. Lyon, & N. A. Krasnegor (Eds.), *Attention, memory, and executive function* (pp. pp. 307–326). Baltimore, MD: Paul H. Brookes.

Barnett, D., Manly, J. T., & Cicchetti, D. (1993). Defining child maltreatment: The interface between policy and research. *Child Abuse, Child Development, and Social Policy*, *8*, 7–73.

Belsky, J., Melhuish, E., Barnes, J., Leyland, A. H., & Romaniuk, H. (2006). Effects of Sure Start local programmes on children and families: Early findings from a quasi-experimental, cross sectional study. *British Medical Journal*, *332*(7556), 1476–1481. doi:10.1136/bmj.38853.451748.2F

Bernier, A., Carlson, S. M., & Whipple, N. (2010). From external regulation to self-regulation: Early parenting precursors of young children's executive functioning. *Child Development*, *81*(1), 326–339. doi:10.1111/cdev.2010.81.issue-1

Bierman, K. L., Nix, R. L., Greenberg, M. T., Blair, C., & Domitrovich, C. E. (2008). Executive functions and school readiness intervention: Impact, moderation, and mediation in the Head Start REDI program. *Development and Psychopathology*, *20*(03), 821–843. doi:10.1017/S0954579408000394

Campbell, S. B., Shaw, D. S., & Gilliom, M. (2000). Early externalizing behavior problems: Toddlers and preschoolers at risk for later maladjustment. *Development and Psychopathology*, *12*(3), 467–488. doi:10.1017/S0954579400003114

Cecil, C. A., Viding, E., Fearon, P., Glaser, D., & McCrory, E. J. (2017). Disentangling the mental health impact of childhood abuse and neglect. *Child Abuse & Neglect*, *63*, 106–119. doi:10.1016/j.chiabu.2016.11.024

Cyr, K., Chamberland, C., Lessard, G., Clément, M. È., Wemmers, J. A., Collin-Vézina, D., … Damant, D. (2012). Polyvictimization in a child welfare sample of children and youths. *Psychology of Violence*, *2*(4), 385–400. doi:10.1037/a0028040

Diamond, A., & Lee, K. (2011). Interventions shown to aid executive function development in children 4 to 12 years old. *Science*, *333*(6045), 959–964. doi:10.1126/science.1204529

Fay-Stammbach, T., Hawes, D. J., & Meredith, P. (2014). Parenting influences on executive function in early childhood: A review. *Child Development Perspectives*, *8*(4), 258–264. doi:10.1111/cdep.2014.8.issue-4

Finkelhor, D., Turner, H., Hamby, S. L., & Ormrod, R. (2011). Polyvictimization: Children's exposure to multiple types of violence, crime, and abuse. *National Survey of Children's Exposure to Violence*. Office of Juvenile Justice and Delinquency Prevention, US Department of Justice, Washington, DC.

Fisher, P. A., Gunnar, M. R., Chamberlain, P., & Reid, J. B. (2000). Preventive intervention for maltreated preschool children: Impact on children's behavior, neuroendocrine activity, and foster parent functioning. *Journal of the American Academy of Child & Adolescent Psychiatry*, *39*(11), 1356–1364. doi:10.1097/00004583-200011000-00009

Fleckman, J. M., Drury, S. S., Taylor, C. A., & Theall, K. P. (2016). Role of direct and indirect violence exposure on externalizing behavior in children. *Journal of Urban Health*, *93*(3), 479–492. doi:10.1007/s11524-016-0052-y

Garon, N., Bryson, S. E., & Smith, I. M. (2008). Executive function in preschoolers: A review using an integrative framework. *Psychological Bulletin, 134*(1), 31–60. doi:10.1037/0033-2909.134.1.31

Gershon, R. C., Wagster, M. V., Hendrie, H. C., Fox, N. A., Cook, K. F., & Nowinski, C. J. (2013). NIH toolbox for assessment of neurological and behavioral function. *Neurology, 80* (11 Supplement 3), S2–S6. doi:10.1212/WNL.0b013e3182872e5f

Greeson, J. K., Briggs, E. C., Kisiel, C. L., Layne, C. M., Ake, G. S., III, Ko, S. J., . . . Fairbank, J. A. (2011). Complex trauma and mental health in children and adolescents placed in foster care: Findings from the National Child Traumatic Stress Network. *Child Welfare, 90*(6), 91–108.

Hayes, A. F. (2013). *Introduction to mediation, moderation, and conditional process analysis: A regression-based approach.* New York, NY: Guilford Press.

Jones, D. J., Lewis, T., Litrownik, A., Thompson, R., Proctor, L. J., Isbell, P., . . . Runyan, D. (2013). Linking childhood sexual abuse and early adolescent risk behavior: The intervening role of internalizing and externalizing problems. *Journal of Abnormal Child Psychology, 41* (1), 139–150. doi:10.1007/s10802-012-9656-1

Kane, M., & Engle, R. (2003). Working-memory capacity and the control of attention: The contributions of goal neglect, response competition, and task set to Stroop interference. *Journal of Experimental Psychology: General, 132*(1), 47–70. doi:10.1037/0096-3445.132.1.47

Keenan, K., & Wakschlag, L. S. (2004). Are oppositional defiant and conduct disorder symptoms normative behaviors in preschoolers? A comparison of referred and nonreferred children. *American Journal of Psychiatry, 161*(2), 356–358. doi:10.1176/appi.ajp.161.2.356

Keil, V., & Price, J. M. (2006). Externalizing behavior disorders in child welfare settings: Definition, prevalence, and implications for assessment and treatment. *Children and Youth Services Review, 28*(7), 761–779. doi:10.1016/j.childyouth.2005.08.006

Kim, J., & Cicchetti, D. (2010). Longitudinal pathways linking child maltreatment, emotion regulation, peer relations, and psychopathology. *Journal of Child Psychology and Psychiatry, 51*(6), 706–716. doi:10.1111/j.1469-7610.2009.02202.x

Klenberg, L., Korkman, M., & Lahti-Nuuttila, P. (2001). Differential development of attention and executive functions in 3-to 12-year-old Finnish children. *Developmental Neuropsychology, 20*(1), 407–428. doi:10.1207/S15326942DN2001_6

Kochanska, G., Murray, K. T., & Harlan, E. T. (2000). Effortful control in early childhood: Continuity and change, antecedents, and implications for social development. *Developmental Psychology, 36*(2), 220–232. doi:10.1037/0012-1649.36.2.220

Korkman, M., Kemp, S., & Kirk, U. (1998). *NEPSY: A developmental neuropsychological assessment.* San Antonio, TX: Psychological Corporation.

Lansford, J. E., Dodge, K. A., Pettit, G. S., Bates, J. E., Crozier, J., & Kaplow, J. (2002). A 12-year prospective study of the long-term effects of early child physical maltreatment on psychological, behavioral, and academic problems in adolescence. *Archives of Pediatrics & Adolescent Medicine, 156*(8), 824–830. doi:10.1001/archpedi.156.8.824

Lansford, J. E., Malone, P. S., Stevens, K. I., Dodge, K. A., Bates, J. E., & Pettit, G. S. (2006). Developmental trajectories of externalizing and internalizing behaviors: Factors underlying resilience in physically abused children. *Development and Psychopathology, 18*(1), 35–55. doi:10.1017/S0954579406060032

Lau, A. S., Leeb, R. T., English, D., Graham, J. C., Briggs, E. C., Brody, K. E., & Marshall, J. M. (2005). What's in a name? A comparison of methods for classifying predominant type of maltreatment. *Child Abuse & Neglect, 29*(5), 533–551. doi:10.1016/j.chiabu.2003.05.005

Leeb, R. T., Lewis, T., & Zolotor, A. J. (2011). A review of physical and mental health consequences of child abuse and neglect and implications for practice. *American Journal of Lifestyle Medicine, 5.5*, 454–468. doi:10.1177/1559827611410266

Manly, J. T., Kim, J. E., Rogosch, F. A., & Cicchetti, D. (2001). Dimensions of child maltreatment and children's adjustment: Contributions of developmental timing and subtype. *Development and Psychopathology, 13*(04), 759–782.

Masten, A. S. (2001). Ordinary magic: Resilience processes in development. *American Psychologist, 56*(3), 227. doi:10.1037/0003-066X.56.3.227

Miller, S. E., & Marcovitch, S. (2015). Examining executive function in the second year of life: Coherence, stability, and relations to joint attention and language. *Developmental Psychology, 51*(1), 101–114. doi:10.1037/a0038359

Moylan, C. A., Herrenkohl, T. I., Sousa, C., Tajima, E. A., Herrenkohl, R. C., & Russo, M. J. (2010). The effects of child abuse and exposure to domestic violence on adolescent internalizing and externalizing behavior problems. *Journal of Family Violence, 25*(1), 53–63. doi:10.1007/s10896-009-9269-9

Obradović, J. (2010). Effortful control and adaptive functioning of homeless children: Variable-focused and person-focused analyses. *Journal of Applied Developmental Psychology, 31*(2), 109–117. doi:10.1016/j.appdev.2009.09.004

Olson, S. L., Tardif, T. Z., Miller, A., Felt, B., Grabell, A. S., Kessler, D., … Hirabayashi, H. (2011). Inhibitory control and harsh discipline as predictors of externalizing problems in young children: A comparative study of US, Chinese, and Japanese preschoolers. *Journal of Abnormal Child Psychology, 39*(8), 1163–1175. doi:10.1007/s10802-011-9531-5

Patterson, G. R., & Yoerger, K. (2002). A developmental model for early-and late-onset delinquency. In J. B. Reid, J. Snyder, & G. R. Patterson (Eds.), *Antisocial behavior in children and adolescents: A developmental analysis and model for intervention* (pp. pp. 147–172). Washington, DC: American Psychological Association.

Pears, K. C., Fisher, P. A., Kim, H. K., Bruce, J., Healey, C. V., & Yoerger, K. (2013). Immediate effects of a school readiness intervention for children in foster care. *Early Education & Development, 24*(6), 771–791. doi:10.1080/10409289.2013.736037

Pears, K. C., Kim, H. K., & Fisher, P. A. (2008). Psychosocial and cognitive functioning of children with specific profiles of maltreatment. *Child Abuse & Neglect, 32*(10), 958–971. doi:10.1016/j.chiabu.2007.12.009

Roman, G. D., Ensor, R., & Hughes, C. (2016). Does executive function mediate the path from mothers' depressive symptoms to young children's problem behaviors? *Journal of Experimental Child Psychology, 142*, 158–170. doi:10.1016/j.jecp.2015.09.022

Roos, L. E., Kim, H. K., Schnabler, S., & Fisher, P. A. (2016). Children's executive function in a CPS-involved sample: Effects of cumulative adversity and specific types of adversity. *Children and Youth Services Review, 71*, 184–190. doi:10.1016/j.childyouth.2016.11.008

Schoemaker, K., Mulder, H., Deković, M., & Matthys, W. (2013). Executive functions in preschool children with externalizing behavior problems: A meta-analysis. *Journal of Abnormal Child Psychology, 41*(3), 457–471. doi:10.1007/s10802-012-9684-x

Slade, E. P., & Wissow, L. S. (2007). The influence of childhood maltreatment on adolescents' academic performance. *Economics of Education Review, 26*(5), 604–614. doi:10.1016/j.econedurev.2006.10.003

Spinrad, T. L., Eisenberg, N., Gaertner, B., Popp, T., Smith, C. L., Kupfer, A., … Hofer, C. (2007). Relations of maternal socialization and toddlers' effortful control to children's adjustment and social competence. *Developmental Psychology, 43*(5), 1170–1186. doi:10.1037/0012-1649.43.5.1170

Stein, E., Evans, B., Mazumdar, R., & Rae-Grant, N. (1996). The mental health of children in foster care: A comparison with community and clinical samples. *The Canadian Journal of Psychiatry*, *41*(6), 385–391. doi:10.1177/070674379604100610

Stormont, M. (2002). Externalizing behavior problems in young children: Contributing factors and early intervention. *Psychology in the Schools*, *39*(2), 127–138. doi:10.1002/(ISSN)1520-6807

Stovall-Mcclough, K. C., & Dozier, M. (2004). Forming attachments in foster care: Infant attachment behaviors during the first 2 months of placement. *Development and Psychopathology*, *16*(02), 253–271. doi:10.1017/S0954579404044505

Sulik, M. J., Blair, C., Mills-Koonce, R., Berry, D., & Greenberg, M. (2015). Early parenting and the development of externalizing behavior problems: Longitudinal mediation through children's executive function. *Child Development*, *86*(5), 1588–1603. doi:10.1111/cdev.2015.86.issue-5

Thorell, L. B., & Wåhlstedt, C. (2006). Executive functioning deficits in relation to symptoms of ADHD and/or ODD in preschool children. *Infant and Child Development*, *15*(5), 503–518. doi:10.1002/(ISSN)1522-7219

Turner, H. A., Finkelhor, D., & Ormrod, R. (2010). Poly-victimization in a national sample of children and youth. *American Journal of Preventive Medicine*, *38*(3), 323–330. doi:10.1016/j.amepre.2009.11.012

3 PTSD and dissociation symptoms as mediators of the relationship between polyvictimization and psychosocial and behavioral problems among justice-involved adolescents

Julian D. Ford, Ruby Charak, Crosby A. Modrowski, and Patricia K. Kerig

ABSTRACT

Polyvictimization (PV) has been shown to be associated with psychosocial and behavioral impairment in community and high risk populations, including youth involved in juvenile justice. However, the mechanisms accounting for these adverse outcomes have not been empirically delineated. Symptoms of post-traumatic stress disorder (PTSD) and dissociation are documented sequelae of PV and are associated with a wide range of behavioral/emotional problems. This study used a cross-sectional research design and bootstrapped multiple mediation analyses with self-report measures completed by a large sample of justice-involved youth (N = 809, ages 12–19 years old, 27% female, 46.5% youth of color) to test the hypothesis that PTSD and dissociation symptoms mediate the relationship between PV and problems with anger, depression/anxiety, alcohol/drug use, and somatic complaints after controlling for the effects of exposure to violence and adversities related to juvenile justice involvement. As hypothesized, PTSD symptoms mediated the relationship of PV with all outcomes except alcohol/drug use problems (which had an unmediated direct association with PV). Partially supporting study hypotheses, dissociation symptoms mediated the relationship between PV and internalizing problems (i.e., depression anxiety; suicide ideation). Implications are discussed for prospective research demarcating the mechanisms linking PV and adverse outcomes in juvenile justice and other high risk populations.

As many as two in three adolescents in the United States report having been exposed to psychological trauma, including victimization experiences that involve directly undergoing or witnessing violence or maltreatment in their family, peer group, school, or community (McLaughlin et al., 2013). Youth who experience multiple *types* of traumatic victimization are at risk for not only PTSD but a complex constellation of biopsychosocial and behavioral problems (Finkelhor, Ormrod, & Turner, 2007; Ford, Connor, & Hawke, 2009; Ford, Elhai, Connor, & Frueh, 2010; Ford, Wasser, & Connor, 2011; Turner, Finkelhor, & Ormrod, 2010), including debilitating anxiety, depression, impulsivity, reactive aggression, social isolation, relational instability and conflict, addictions, delinquency, physical health problems and risks, and educational and developmental delays (D'Andrea, Ford, Stolbach, Spinazzola, & Van Der Kolk, 2012; Ford, 2017; Ford & Gomez, 2015; Le, Holton, Romero, & Fisher, 2016).

Polyvictimization (PV) overlaps with, but is distinct from, other concepts that have been developed to account for the burden on health and development. For example, allostatic load (McEwen & Lasley, 2003), is a term used to describe the physiological burden that accumulates when children are exposed to multiple types of traumatic stressors or victimization (D. Grasso, Greene, & Ford, 2013). Additionally, the constructs of cumulative trauma (Cloitre et al., 2009), adverse childhood experiences (ACE) (Anda, Butchart, Felitti, & Brown, 2010), and complex or developmental trauma (D'Andrea et al., 2012) have been empirically demonstrated to have robust relationships with biopsychosocial impairments across the lifespan. ACEs refer to the incremental adverse impact of experiencing one or more forms of maltreatment, violence, and impaired caregivers in childhood. Similarly, complex/developmental trauma refers to exposure to intentional acts of maltreatment, victimization or losses as a witness or directly, sensitive periods of development including adulthood, as well as childhood. Cumulative trauma refers to exposure to multiple types of potentially traumatic stressors, including non-interpersonal (e.g., severe accidents or disasters), as well as interpersonal (e.g., maltreatment, violence) forms of trauma.

PV similarly involves exposure to *multiple types* of potentially traumatic events or adverse interpersonal experiences, but instead of progressively increasing risk trajectories postulated by the cumulative and complex/developmental trauma and ACE paradigms, PV posits a categorical *threshold* formulation: risk of severe impairment is predicted to take a quantum leap when a defined dose of different types of victimization (i.e., the threshold) has been exceeded. Similar to the complex trauma model, PV also does not limit the types of victimization to events that meet the PTSD criterion for traumatic stressors, as does the cumulative trauma model, nor to the specific types of maltreatment, violence, and caregiver impairment identified by the ACE framework.

However, the PV construct is subject to a limitation that is problematic for the cumulative trauma, complex/developmental trauma, and ACE paradigms as well. Counting each discrete type of victimization, trauma, or adversity as equivalent to all other types fails to address the possibility that different types of victimization, trauma, or adversity may have non-equal impacts on risk and impairment (McLaughlin & Sheridan, 2016). Recognition of this issue has resulted in a modified operational definition of lifetime PV that weights childhood maltreatment and sexual assault four and three times greater, respectively, than all other forms of victimization (Finkelhor, Ormrod, & Turner, 2009). Nevertheless, those weightings still equate the relative contribution of all other types of victimization, and cannot be assumed to accurately represent each victimization type's relative risk across a variety of age groups and populations.

An alternative to this *a priori* approach to defining and categorizing PV is the person-centered method of empirically identifying distinct profiles of types of victimization, without assuming *a priori* the relative contribution of each type to the individual's risk of impairment (Ford et al., 2010). Using this approach, several recent studies have found similar PV profiles among youth that are consistently associated with the most severe psychosocial and legal problems despite being characterized by different types and probabilities of victimization (Adams et al., 2016; Aebi et al., 2015; Ballard et al., 2015; Burns, Lagdon, Boyda, & Armour, 2016; Charak et al., 2016; Ford, Grasso, Hawke, & Chapman, 2013; French, Bi, Latimore, Klemp, & Butler, 2014; D. J. Grasso, Dierkhising, Branson, Ford, & Lee, 2015; Turner, Shattuck, Finkelhor, & Hamby, 2016).

Two of the person-centered studies of PV conducted to date involved a sub-population of adolescents at high risk for victimization: youth involved in the juvenile justice system (Aebi et al., 2015; Ford et al., 2013). Psychological trauma and posttraumatic stress disorder (PTSD) are 3–8 times more prevalent among youth involved in the juvenile justice system (Abram et al., 2004; Adams et al., 2013; Ford, Hartman, Hawke, & Chapman, 2008; Leibowitz, Laser, & Burton, 2011) compared to youth in the community (McLaughlin et al., 2013). Even in this highly trauma-affected sub-population, a distinct subset of between 5–65% of justice-involved youth have been identified as polyvictims and shown to have more severe psychosocial problems than other trauma-exposed youth in the justice system (DeHart & Moran, 2015; Ford et al., 2013; Pereda, Abad, & Guilera, 2015; Segura, Pereda, Guilera, & Abad, 2016). Youth in the community who have been polyvictimized also have been found to be at elevated risk for delinquency and juvenile justice involvement (Ford et al., 2013; D. J. Grasso et al., 2015). Recent research also has been devoted to identifying the mechanisms linking PV to youth involvement in the justice system. A number of potential pathways from victimization to juvenile justice involvement have been identified (Ford, Chapman, Mack, & Pearson, 2006), as well as from childhood adversity to PV (Finkelhor, Ormrod, Turner, & Holt, 2009). However, the pathways linking PV to biopsychosocial impairment have not been systematically investigated. A recent research review recommended focusing on the identification of mechanisms linking childhood adversity and psychopathology outcomes, identifying disrupted emotional processing and poor executive function as potential key mechanisms (McLaughlin, 2016).

The present report therefore addresses the question of whether PV's association with youth maladaptation is mediated by disruptions in emotion processing and executive function, with PTSD and dissociation symptoms serving as proxies for these potential mechanisms. PTSD has been found to be associated with PV in adolescents (Ford et al., 2010), and specifically in juvenile justice-involved youth (Ford et al., 2013). Variants of PV, including complex trauma (Van Dijke, Ford, Frank, & Van Der Hart, 2015) and developmental trauma (D'Andrea et al., 2012) have been shown to be associated with severe dissociation in youth and adults, and specifically among incarcerated girls (McReynolds & Wasserman, 2011). Moreover, PTSD has been conceptualized as fundamentally involving disruptions in emotion processing (Rauch & Foa, 2006; Southwick et al., 2003) and executive function (Olff, Polak, Witteveen, & Denys, 2014). Pathological dissociation has been postulated to be a marker for severe emotion dysregulation (Ford, 2009), and to be a cognitive processing style (Dorahy, 2006; Lanius, 2015) that is associated with impaired executive function (Rivera-Velez, Gonzalez-Viruet, Martinez-Taboas, & Perez-Mojica, 2014); alterations in executive function may be a risk factor along with exposure to family violence for dissociative problems in childhood (DePrince, Weinzierl, & Combs, 2008). Therefore, consistent with McLaughlin's (2016) multifinality conceptualization, the relationship between PV and internalizing and externalizing problems among justice-involved youth was *hypothesized to be mediated by symptoms of PTSD and dissociation.*

The present report extends the results of previously reported latent class analyses which identified three sub-groups in a sample of justice-involved youth who reported, on average, more than 10 (of 26 possible) types of potentially traumatic events (PTEs) in their lifetimes (Authors, in review). A *Mixed adversity (MA)* class (41% of the sample) relatively infrequently reported PTEs, but more than 40% of these youths reported a variety of adversities including a parent arrested or someone they knew attempted suicide, severely injury or illness, or physical abuse. A *Violent environment (VE)* class (41% of the sample) was characterized by frequent (64–91%) reporting of physical abuse or assault, severe injury or illness, witnessing physical assaults or a parent using drugs, or someone close attempting or committing suicide or being violently injured or killed. A PV class (18% of the sample) was characterized by frequent (80–90%) reporting of each of 10 types of victimization (sexual abuse, physical abuse or assault, emotional abuse, having a parent threaten to leave them, witnessing physical assaults, and the unexpected death or attempted suicide of someone they knew). More than half of the youth in the poly-victim class also reported witnessing inter-parental or family violence, having a parent arrested, being removed from or abandoned by their parents, and having a loved one violently injured or killed.

Consistent with prior studies with justice-involved youths (Ford et al., 2013, 2008), the polyvictim sub-group in this sample had more severe depression and anxiety, somatic distress, and suicidality, alcohol or drug use, and anger/irritability symptoms than the MA sub-group (Authors, in review). They also had more severe depression and anxiety, somatic distress, and suicidality symptoms than the VE class. The VE sub-group reported intermediate levels of severity on all symptom measures, and significantly more severe alcohol or drug use, and anger/irritability symptoms than the MA sub-group. In order to extend these findings, the current report tested the comparative hypothesis that PTSD and dissociation symptoms would uniquely mediate the relationship between polyvictimization and youth maladaptation after controlling for the effects of (a) exposure to violence in the family and community, and (b) MAs related to involvement in juvenile justice.

Method

Participants

Participants were 809 youth (210 girls, 599 boys) recruited from a short-term juvenile detention center located in the western United States. On average, youth were 16.08 years old (SD = 1.30, range 12–19 years old). The sample was ethnically diverse and was consistent with the ethnic composition of the justice-involved population of the geographic region. Specifically, 53.6% were White/Caucasian, 25.8% Hispanic/Latino, 5.7% multi-racial, 3.8% Pacific Islander/Native Hawaiian, 4.9% Black/African American, 3.7% Native American/Alaskan Native, and 0.9% Asian American.

Procedure

All study procedures were approved by both the University of Utah and the State of Utah Department of Human Services Institutional Review Boards. During the detention center's visiting hours, research assistants approached legal guardians and asked if they were interested in participating in the study. Additionally, legal guardians were asked if they would provide permission for a research assistant to approach their child about participating in the study. If the legal guardian was interested in participating in the study, research staff collected signed informed consent. After obtaining informed consent, youth were approached and asked if they would be interested in participating in the study. If youths were interested in participating, they provided signed assent and completed study measures on a laptop computer in a private room at the detention center. In order to protect against any perception of coercion, no incentives were offered for participating in the study.

Measures

Trauma exposure and posttraumatic stress symptoms

Youth completed the UCLA Posttraumatic Stress Disorder Reaction Index—Adolescent Version (PTSD–RI) for *DSM–5* (Steinberg et al., 2013). The first set of questions ask youth about their lifetime exposure to 14 PTEs in accordance with Criterion A. Youth also reported on additional traumatic events, such as prolonged separation from a caregiver or experiences of neglect, that are not categorized as PTEs by the current DSM-5 criteria. The second set of questions on the PTSD-RI asks youth to report on the extent to which they have experienced past-month PTSD symptoms. Items are presented on a Likert scale ranging from 0 (*none of the time*) to 4 (*most of the time*). Symptoms from Criterion B, C, D, and E were summed to calculate a PTSD total score (α = .92), with higher scores representing more severe PTSD symptoms.

Dissociation

Dissociation was measured as a sum of four PTSD-RI items that assess depersonalization and derealization (α = .71); higher scores represent more severe dissociation.

Mental health problems

The Massachusetts Youth Screening Instrument Version 2 (MAYSI-2) (Archer, Simonds-Bisbee, Spiegel, Handel, & Elkins, 2010; Grisso, Barnum, Fletcher, Cauffman, & Peuschold, 2001) is a brief self-report inventory designed specifically for use in juvenile detention centers that screens for a wide range of potential mental health problems. The MAYSI-2 is meant to be administered to youth by detention center staff within 24–48 hours of admission to a detention facility. The current study utilized the following scales: alcohol/drug use (α = .84), anger-irritability (α = .81), depressed/anxious (α = .75), somatic complaints (α = .79), and suicide ideation (α = .88).

Statistical analyses

Bivariate correlations were first conducted to test the association between PTSD and dissociation symptom severity and MAYSI-2 scale scores (alcohol/drug use, anger/irritability, depression/anxiety, somatic complaints, and suicide ideation). All descriptive analyses, dummy coding and bivariate correlations were analyzed in IBM SPSS version 23.

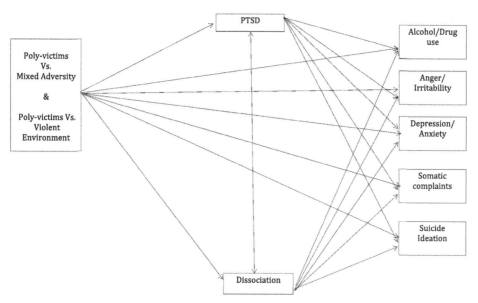

Figure 1. Hypothesized direct and mediated pathways between Poly-victimization Class (versus Violent Environment Class and Mixed Adversity Class) and internalizing and externalizing mental health problems, with PTSD symptoms and dissociation as mediators. Note: All error terms of the mental health outcomes are intercorrelated.

Second, the three sub-groups previously identified via a latent class analysis were dummy-coded in a mediation model (Figure 1) using IBM-SPSS. The model designated the Polyvictim (PV) class as reference group (coded 0), comparing it to the MA and VE classes. Using M*plus* version 7. 31 (Muthén & Muthén, 2015), mediation analysis was carried out to evaluate the indirect effects of class-membership (PV vs. MA and PV vs. VE), on the dependent variables, the MAYSI-2 A/D, A/I, D/A, SA, and SI scales, through the mediating variables of PTSD and dissociation symptom severity. Multiple mediation analysis is an extension of simple mediation in which the separate and combined mediation of two or more mediators is simultaneously modeled (Preacher & Hayes, 2008). All variables were treated as manifest/observed variables. Bivariate correlations were calculated between the error terms for PTSD and dissociation symptoms, and among the MAYSI-2 scales. The magnitude of the indirect effects was examined using the product-of-coefficient approach (Bishop, Fienberg, & Holland, 1975) to calculate standard errors of the indirect effects. The coefficient of the indirect effect is divided by its standard error and compared to a critical value with a z-test. As recommended by Preacher and Hayes (2008), bias-corrected bootstrapping procedures for confidence intervals with a total of 5,000 bootstrapped samples were used to corroborate findings from the product-of-coefficient tests. Use of bootstrapping method is recommended over the traditional causal steps approach, as the former has higher power while maintaining reasonable control over the Type I error rate (MacKinnon, Lockwood, & Williams, 2004). In the

Table 1. Correlations of PTSD, dissociation, and internalizing and externalizing symptoms

Variables	Dissociation	A/D U	A/I	D/A	SC	SI
PTSD Symptoms	.64***	.16***	.33***	.46***	.35***	.28***
Dissociation		.11**	.26***	.49***	.27***	.25***
Alcohol/Drug Use (AD/U)			.35***	.18***	.26***	.14***
Anger/Irritability (A/I)				.61***	.49***	.41***
Depression/Anxiety (D/A)					.58***	.63***
Somatic Complaints (SC)						.39***

Note: PTSD = posttraumatic stress disorder
***p < .001

present study, a 95% confidence interval not containing a zero was considered statistically significant. Third, all significant specific indirect effects for PTSD and dissociations symptoms were compared with each other, with the Model constraint option in M*plus* that calculates a Wald test to examine differences between parameters under consideration (each pair of statistically significant indirect effects) using bootstrapping (*N* = 5,000 iterations).

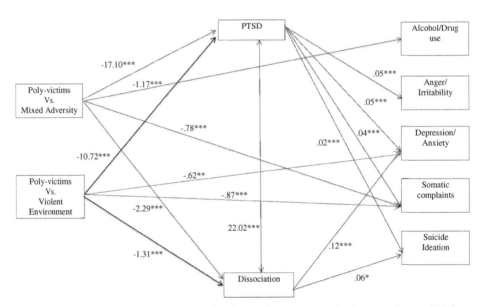

Figure 2. Significant direct and mediated pathways between Mixed Adversity class and Violent Environment classes (versus Poly-victimization) and internalizing and externalizing problems with PTSD and dissociation as mediators.
Note: All error terms of the mental health outcomes are significantly intercorrelated at p < .05.
***p < .001. **p < .01. *p < .05.

Table 2. Statistically significant mediation (indirect effects) by PTSD or dissociation of the association of PV class membership (versus MA or VE class membership) with MAYSI-2 scales

Pathways	Indirect effect (B)	Indirect effect 95% CI
PV Class vs. MA Class→PTSD→MAYSI subscales		
1 PV Class vs. MA Class→PTSD→MAYSI-Anger/Irritability	-.82	-1.21, -.47
2 PV Class vs. MA Class→PTSD→MAYSI-Depression/Anxiety	-.84	-1.14, -.59
3 PV Class vs. MA Class→PTSD→MAYSI-Somatic complaints	-.59	-.84, -.32
4 PV Class vs. MA Class→PTSD→MAYSI-Suicide ideation	-.31	-.53, -.13
PV Class vs. MA Class→ Dissociation→MAYSI subscales		
5 PV Class vs. MA Class→Dissociation→MAYSI-Depression/ Anxiety	-.28	-.13, -.50
6 PV Class vs. MA Class→Dissociation→MAYSI-Suicide ideation	-.14	-.29, -.03
PV Class vs. VE Class→PTSD→MAYSI subscales		
7 PV Class vs. VE Class→PTSD →MAYSI-Anger/Irritability	-.51	-.30, -.81
8 PV Class vs. VE Class→PTSD →MAYSI-Depression/anxiety	-.53	-.35, -.76
9 PV Class vs. VE Class→PTSD →MAYSI-Somatic complaints	-.37	-.56, -.20
10 PV Class vs. VE Class→PTSD→MAYSI-Suicide ideation	-.20	-.36, -.08
PV Class vs. VE Class→Dissociation→MAYSI subscales		
11 PV Class vs. VE Class→Dissociation →MAYSI-Depression/ Anxiety	$-.16^{ns}$	-.30, .07
12 PV Class vs. VE Class→Dissociation →MAYSI-Somatic complaints	-.08	-.20, -.01
13 PV Class vs. VE Class→Dissociation →MAYSI-Suicide ideation	-.08	-.18, -.02

Notes: PV = Polyvictimization; MA = Mixed Adversity; VE = Violent Environments; PTSD = posttraumatic stress disorder symptoms; MAYSI = Massachusetts Youth Screening Instrument. Superscript ns denotes $p < .05$.

Results

Bivariate correlations demonstrated that all study variables were statistically significantly correlated (Table 1). Correlations ranged from $r = .11–.16$ with alcohol/drug use to .46–.49 with depression/anxiety, with a median $r = .28$

As shown in Figure 2, PV class membership was associated with higher PTSD and dissociation symptom severity than MA and VE class membership. (The negative valence of these and the direct pathway coefficients indicate that MA and VE class members had lower scores than PV class members.) The only direct (unmediated) pathways to the mental health outcomes involved an association of PV class membership (vs. MA class membership) with higher alcohol/drug use and somatic complaints, and of PV class membership (vs. VE class membership) with more severe depression/ anxiety symptoms and somatic complaints. PTSD symptom severity was directly associated with greater severity of most outcome variables; the only exception was alcohol/drug use. Dissociation symptom severity was directly associated only with severity of depression/anxiety symptoms and suicide ideation.

Table 3. Pairwise comparison of the strength of statistically significant indirect effects.

Indirect effects	Estimate	95% CI
PV Class vs. MA Class→PTSD→MAYSI subscales		
Anger/Irritability vs. Depression/Anxiety	.02	-.27, .31
Anger/Irritability vs. Somatic Complaints	-.22	-.55, .10
Anger/Irritability vs. Suicide Ideation	**-.50**	-.83, -.19
Depression/Anxiety vs. Somatic Complaints	**-.25**	-.52, -.03
Depression/Anxiety vs. Suicide Ideation	**-.53**	-.77, -.32
Somatic Complaints vs. Suicide Ideation	**-.28**	-.53, -.06
PV Class vs. MA Class→Dissociation→ MAYSI subscales		
Depression/Anxiety vs. Suicide Ideation	**-.14**	-.30 to -.01
PV Class vs. VE Class→PTSD→MAYSI subscales		
Anger/Irritability vs. Depression/Anxiety	.02	-.18, .20
Anger/Irritability vs. Somatic Complaints	-.14	-.36, .06
Anger/Irritability vs. Suicide Ideation	**-.32**	-.55, -.12
Depression/Anxiety vs. Somatic Complaints	**-.15**	-.34, -.02
Depression/Anxiety vs. Suicide Ideation	**-.33**	-.49, -.20
Somatic Complaints vs. Suicide Ideation	**-.18**	-.34, -.01
PV Class vs. VE Class→Dissociation→MAYSI subscales		
Depression/Anxiety vs. Suicide Ideation	**-.08**	-.20, -.01

Notes: PV = Polyvictimization; MA = Mixed Adversity; VE = Violent Environments; PTSD = posttraumatic stress disorder symptoms; MAYSI = Massachusetts Youth Screening Instrument; Estimates in **bold** font are $p < .05$.

Consistent with the path model results, mediation by PTSD was statistically significant in the relationship between PV class membership (vs. VE or MA class membership) and more severe anger /irritability, depression/anxiety symptoms, somatic complaints, and suicide ideation (Table 2). Dissociation also significantly mediated relationships between PV class membership (versus VE or MA class membership) with more severe problems, but only with internalizing (i.e., depression/anxiety symptoms; suicide ideation) and not externalizing problems (Table 2).

Finally, analyses examining the relative strength of the indirect/mediation effects of PTSD and dissociation symptoms for different MAYSI-2 internalizing and externalizing problem variables were conducted. For the unique relationship between PV and the outcome variables (i.e., comparisons of PV vs. *both* VE and MA; see Table 3), PTSD symptoms had a significantly stronger indirect (mediation) effect for depression/anxiety and anger/irritability than for suicide ideation, and for depression/anxiety than for somatic complaints. Dissociation symptoms had a significantly stronger indirect (mediation) effect for depression/anxiety than for suicide ideation (again for *both* the PV vs. VE and MA comparisons; Table 3).

Discussion

As hypothesized, PTSD symptoms mediated the relationship of PV with most of the adverse mental health outcomes, and the only exception (alcohol/drug use problems) had an unmediated direct association with PV. Partially supporting study hypotheses, dissociation symptoms mediated the relationship between PV and internalizing problems (i.e., depression anxiety; suicide ideation), but not with externalizing problems (i.e., anger/irritability; alcohol/drug. Study findings thus suggest that both PTSD and dissociation symptoms may play roles – albeit not identically – in the association of PV with emotional, behavioral, and physical health problems among justice-involved youth. The relation of these findings to prior research and their implications for future research and clinical practice will be discussed.

The finding that PTSD symptoms mediated PV's association with several types of internalizing psychopathology is consistent with evidence that by PTSD symptoms are one of several interrelated internalizing sequelae of PV (Ford et al., 2010, 2013; Voisin, Hotton, Schneider, & Team, 2017). It also suggests that PTSD may be a unique pathway from PV to a wide range of internalizing problems, which could provide a focus for targeted psychotherapy for traumatized youth who present with an often complex array of psychosocial symptoms (D'Andrea et al., 2012). These symptoms include not only dysphoria but also potentially debilitating or life-threatening physical health problems (Ballard et al., 2015; Ford et al., 2013; Lee, 2015; Miller-Graff, Cater, Howell, & Graham-Bermann, 2015; Radatz & Wright, 2015; Seng, D'Andrea, & Ford, 2014; Soler, Segura, Kirchner, & Forns, 2013; Stansfeld et al., 2016; Thompson et al., 2015; Turner, Finkelhor, Shattuck, & Hamby, 2012; Widom, Horan, & Brzustowicz, 2015) and suicidality (Charak et al., 2016).

PTSD symptoms also may be a link between PV and youths' externalizing problems, which is particularly relevant in the population of youth in or at risk for involvement in juvenile justice (Ford et al., 2012). The link to from PV to PTSD symptoms and ultimately to externalizing problems was clearest in this study in problems with anger/irritability (Charak et al., 2016; Cudmore, Cuevas, & Sabina, 2015; Cuevas, Finkelhor, Clifford, Ormrod, & Turner, 2010; Hamby, Finkelhor, & Turner, 2013; Maneta, Cohen, Schulz, & Waldinger, 2012; Messman-Moore, Walsh, & Dilillo, 2010). Thus, emotion dysregulation in the form of difficulty with anger may occur as a downstream effect of PV -related PTSD symptoms, and this may lead to not only externalizing behavior problems and delinquency (Ford et al., 2010) but also suicide risk (Charak et al., 2016) and additional re-victimization (Cuevas et al., 2010; Finkelhor et al., 2009; Messman-Moore et al., 2010).

Dissociation symptoms also had indirect effects, but only for the relationships between PV and internalizing problems involving dysphoria (i.e., depression/anxiety and suicide ideation). This is consistent with research that has identified a sub-group of individuals with histories of childhood sexual abuse and other interpersonal traumas who are characterized by comorbid depression and dissociative symptoms (Bohn, Bernardy, Wolfe, & Hauser, 2013; Dorahy et al., 2013; Sar, Akyuz, Ozturk, & Alioglu, 2013; Seng et al., 2014), and who are at risk for suicidality (Foote, Smolin, Neft, & Lipschitz, 2008; Ford & Gomez, 2015; Sar et al., 2013; Tamar-Gurol, Sar, Karadag, Evren, & Karagoz, 2008). Comorbid depression and dissociation following exposure to interpersonal trauma also may involve a complex combination of memory disruptions (Gagnon, Lee, & DePrince, 2017), executive function impairments (Bruce, Ray, Bruce, Arnett, & Carlson, 2007; DePrince et al., 2008; Li et al., 2013; Rivera-Velez et al., 2014), self-blame (Babcock & DePrince, 2012), and somatic problems (Kilic et al., 2014; Scioli-Salter et al., 2016) – that are related to, but distinct from, PTSD (Collin-Vezina & Hebert, 2005).

Alcohol and drug use problems, by contrast, were not associated with either PTSD or dissociation symptoms, but were directly related to PV (compared to multiple adversity class membership). This is consistent with reports of a relationship between PV and substance use problems (Chan, 2015; Cornelius et al., 2010; Danielson et al., 2010; Fite et al., 2016; Ford et al., 2010, 2008; Lucenko, Sharkova, Huber, Jemelka, & Mancuso, 2015; Wade et al., 2016). PV also may be a negative prognostic factor for adolescent substance abuse treatment (Shane, Diamond, Mensinger, Shera, & Wintersteen, 2006). Disentangling the potential contributions to substance use problems of direct victimization versus living in a family or community in which trauma and substance abuse have been historically prevalent remains an important area for investigation and careful clinical assessment (Ehlers, Gizer, Gilder, Ellingson, & Yehuda, 2013; Estrada, 2009; Kelley et al., 2010; Myhra, 2011; Perron, Gotham, & Cho, 2008).

Somatic problems, in turn, were related to PV both independently of PTSD and dissociation symptoms, as well as via an indirect relationship mediated by PTSD symptoms. This finding is consistent with prior reports of a relationship between PV or ACE and physical health problems in childhood, adolescence, and adulthood (Chartier, Walker, & Naimark, 2010; Ford et al., 2013; Miller-Graff et al., 2015; Ramiro, Madrid, & Brown, 2010; Slopen, McLaughlin, Dunn, & Koenen, 2013; Voisin, Bird, Shiu, & Krieger, 2013). The association for PV occurred over and above the effects of living in a VE, suggest that childhood maltreatment and traumatically disrupted family and caregiving relationships may cause particularly insidious harm to children's physical health and body development – consistent with the allostatic load (McEwen & Lasley, 2003) and developmental trauma disorder (D'Andrea et al., 2012; Ford et al., 2013) paradigms.

The indirect effects of both PTSD and dissociation symptoms were strongest for the depression/anxiety outcome variable, and secondarily for the anger/irritability and somatic complaints outcome variables. This may be in part due to the substantial overlap between PTSD and depression/anxiety symptoms (Ford, Elhai, Ruggiero, & Frueh, 2009; McCullagh, Quinn, Voisin, & Schneider, 2017). However, anger and somatic problems are also primary PTSD symptoms, so this suggests that emotion dysregulation involving dysphoria and fear may be a primary maladaptive trajectory for polyvictimized youth in juvenile justice. Dissociation may be involved in that maladaptive trajectory when emotion dysregulation becomes sufficiently severe to alter cognitive/executive function (Ford, 2009) – consistent with the potential mediating role of dissociation identified in the relationship between childhood sexual abuse and self-injury amongst youth involved in juvenile justice (Chaplo, Kerig, Bennett, & Modrowski, 2015).

These findings suggest that identifying youths in juvenile detention who have histories of PV is important in order to ensure that these youths receive thorough assessment and case planning that includes evidence-based trauma-informed clinical and educational services for targeted problems. These include serious safety risks to themselves (e.g., depression or anxiety disorders, alcohol and drug use, suicidal ideation), as well as difficulties that that place youth at risk for costly health problems (i.e., somatic complaints) and for further and increasingly chronic involvement in the juvenile and criminal justice systems (e.g., anger, alcohol and drug use) (Dierkhising & Branson, 2016; Ford, Kerig, Desai, & Feierman, 2016).

A variety of barriers (e.g., limited resources, lack of clarity in defining core concepts and operational procedures, tension between punitive versus restorative approaches to programming) have limited the implementation of trauma-informed services in juvenile justice systems (Branson, Baetz, Horwitz, & Hoagwood, 2017). The sheer number of justice-involved youth who have been victimized precludes providing all of them with specialized milieu and community services, given that as many as 90% have experienced traumatic victimization or severe adversity in childhood. The sub-group of polyvictims (i.e., 18% of the sample in the current study) could feasibly be identified, and provided with evidence-based trauma-specific assessment and therapeutic/rehabilitative interventions (Ford et al., 2016). This could provide a framework for juvenile justice practices and milieus that are safer and more effectively rehabilitative for all justice-involved youths, their families and schools, and for the adult juvenile justice staff and law enforcement personnel in their communities (Ford et al., 2013).

Study findings should be considered in the context of several methodological limitations. The convenience sample of consecutive admissions to juvenile detention centers in a state in the western United States from whom parental/legal guardian consent and youth assent were obtained may not be representative of other juvenile justice populations, However, the samples was relatively ethnoculturally diverse with substantial representation of Hispanic youth and was similar demographically and in legal charges to the overall census of the detention centers during the study period. Missing data ranged from 2.35% to 17.9% on the PTE and other self-report measures. However, there were no differences between the latent classes on the extent of missing data for any measure, and there was no evidence of a non-random pattern of missing trauma. The sub-sample of females was smaller than that of males, which precluded separate analyses for girls and boys in order to test for any gender-specific relationships. In light of the over-representation of girls in the polyvictim class, it will be important to examine the impact of PV on justice-involved girls in future studies.

The cross-sectional and retrospective research design does not permit con-clusions of causality or the temporal sequencing of the relationships between PV and the symptom measures, nor that PTSD or dissociation symptoms actually serve as mediators of those relationships (Kraemer, 2010). Prospective studies that ascertain the longitudinal course of the sequelae of poly-victimization are necessary to confirm mediation (Ouellet-Morin et al., 2015; Widom et al., 2015). The validity of self-report of sensitive matters, such as trauma history, depression, suicidality, and substance use problems by adolescents in the juvenile justice system may be affected by the constraints of the legal context (e.g., reluctance to disclose PTEs or symptoms due to fear of stigma or legal consequences), learning or reading impairments (Jensen, Fabiano, Lopez-Williams, & Chacko, 2006), or dysphoria (Kuyken & Dalgleish, 2011). Justice-involved youth often have had school problems, with reading levels less than their chronological age (Lansing et al., 2014), but nevertheless usually have completed at least the fifth grade and are able to read and (despite threats to validity, such as early post-admission dysphoria and reluctance to admit problems) validly respond to self-report questionnaires (Bennett, Modrowski, Kerig, & Chaplo, 2015; Kerig, Bennett, Thompson, & Becker, 2012) or such as those used in this study. Under-reporting associated with hypervigilance and emotional numbing (Bennett & Kerig, 2014) or with the dissociative sub-type of PTSD (Bennett et al., 2015) may have obscured relationships either between dissociation and outcome variables other than depression and suicidality or between both dissociation and PTSD symptoms with alcohol and drug use problems. Replication is needed before those null relationships can be considered a definite finding, as well as to confirm the indirect effect relationships that were significant in this sample.

In conclusion, study findings suggest that symptoms of PTSD and dissociation may be a link between PV and internalizing problems that can impair the functioning and compromise the safety (e.g., suicidality) and legal status (e.g., anger) of youth involved in the juvenile justice system. PTSD and dissociation symptoms were not only most severe and but also had the strongest indirect effects for polyvictims, compared to other justice-involved youth who had exten-sive histories of undergoing or witnessing violence or who had experienced a lesser (but still often noteworthy) degree of adversity in troubled families or communities. Research is needed to determine if there is a life pathway leading from PV through PTSD and dissociation symptoms to severe emotion dysregulation – which could serve as a basis for targeting the treatment of PTSD and dissociation for this sub-set of troubled youth who have become involved in juvenile justice. The relationship between PV and alcohol and drug use problems with no intermediary relationship through dissociation or PTSD symptoms indicates that other potential mediators or mechanisms also require identification in order to fully demarcate the life pathways between PV and adverse outcomes in this population.

Funding

Preparation of this report was supported by funding from the Substance Abuse and Mental Health Services Administration [1U79SM080044-01] (Center for Trauma Recovery and Juvenile Justice), J. Ford, Principal Investigator. Julian Ford is the co-owner of Advanced Trauma Solutions, Inc., the sole licensed distributor of the TARGET© intervention by the University of Connecticut. No other author reports a potential conflict of interest.

References

Abram, K. M., Teplin, L. A., Charles, D. R., Longworth, S. L., McClelland, G. M., & Dulcan, M. K. (2004). Posttraumatic stress disorder and trauma in youth in juvenile detention. *Archives of General Psychiatry*, *61*(4), 403–410. 61/4/403 [pii]. doi: 10.1001/archpsyc.61.4.403

Adams, Z. W., McCart, M. R., Zajac, K., Danielson, C. K., Sawyer, G. K., Saunders, B. E., & Kilpatrick, D. G. (2013). Psychiatric problems and trauma exposure in nondetained delinquent and nondelinquent adolescents. *Journal of Clinical Child and Adolescent Psychology*, *42*(3), 323–331. doi:10.1080/15374416.2012.749786

Adams, Z. W., Moreland, A., Cohen, J. R., Lee, R. C., Hanson, R. F., Danielson, C. K., … Briggs, E. C. (2016). Polyvictimization: Latent profiles and mental health outcomes in a clinical sample of adolescents. *Psychology of Violence*, *6*(1), 145–155. doi:10.1037/a0039713

Aebi, M., Linhart, S., Thun-Hohenstein, L., Bessler, C., Steinhausen, H. C., & Plattner, B. (2015). Detained male adolescent offender's emotional, physical and sexual maltreatment profiles and their associations to psychiatric disorders and criminal behaviors. *Journal of Abnormal Child Psychology*, *43*(5), 999–1009. doi:10.1007/s10802-014-9961-y

Anda, R. F., Butchart, A., Felitti, V. J., & Brown, D. W. (2010). Building a framework for global surveillance of the public health implications of adverse childhood experiences. *American Journal of Preventive Medicine*, *39*(1), 93–98. S0749-3797(10)00277-1 [pii]. doi: 10.1016/j.amepre.2010.03.015

Archer, R. P., Simonds-Bisbee, E. C., Spiegel, D. R., Handel, R. W., & Elkins, D. E. (2010). Validity of the Massachusetts youth screening instrument-2 (MAYSI-2) scales in juvenile justice settings. *Journal of Personality Assessment*, *92*(4), 337–348. doi:10.1080/00223891.2010.482009

Babcock, R. L., & DePrince, A. P. (2012). Childhood betrayal trauma and self-blame appraisals among survivors of intimate partner abuse. *Journal of Trauma and Dissociation, 13*(5), 526–538. doi:10.1080/15299732.2012.694842

Ballard, E. D., Van Eck, K., Musci, R. J., Hart, S. R., Storr, C. L., Breslau, N., & Wilcox, H. C. (2015). Latent classes of childhood trauma exposure predict the development of behavioral health outcomes in adolescence and young adulthood. *Psychological Medicine, 45*(15), 3305–3316. doi:10.1017/S0033291715001300

Bennett, D. C., & Kerig, P. K. (2014). Investigating the construct of trauma-related acquired callousness among delinquent youth: Differences in emotion processing. *Journal of Traumatic Stress, 27*(4), 415–422. doi:10.1002/jts.21931

Bennett, D. C., Modrowski, C. A., Kerig, P. K., & Chaplo, S. D. (2015). Investigating the dissociative subtype of posttraumatic stress disorder in a sample of traumatized detained youth. *Psychological Trauma : Theory, Research, Practice and Policy, 7*(5), 465–472. doi:10.1037/tra0000057

Bishop, Y. M., Fienberg, S. E., & Holland, P. W. (1975). *Discrete multivariate analysis: Theory and practice.* Cambridge, MA: MIT Press.

Bohn, D., Bernardy, K., Wolfe, F., & Hauser, W. (2013). The association among childhood maltreatment, somatic symptom intensity, depression, and somatoform dissociative symptoms in patients with fibromyalgia syndrome: A single-center cohort study. *Journal of Trauma and Dissociation, 14*(3), 342–358. doi:10.1080/15299732.2012.736930

Branson, C. E., Baetz, C. L., Horwitz, S. M., & Hoagwood, K. E. (2017). Trauma-informed juvenile justice systems: A systematic review of definitions and core components. *Psychological Trauma, 9*(6), 635–646. doi:10.1037/tra0000255

Bruce, A. S., Ray, W. J., Bruce, J. M., Arnett, P. A., & Carlson, R. A. (2007). The relationship between executive functioning and dissociation. *Journal of Clinical and Experimental Neuropsychology, 29*(6), 626–633. doi:10.1080/13803390600878901

Burns, C. R., Lagdon, S., Boyda, D., & Armour, C. (2016). Interpersonal polyvictimization and mental health in males. *Journal of Anxiety Disorders, 40,* 75–82. doi:10.1016/j.janxdis.2016.04.002

Chan, K. L. (2015). Family polyvictimization and elevated levels of addiction and psychopathology among parents in a Chinese household sample. *Journal of Interpersonal Violence.* doi:10.1177/0886260515592617

Chaplo, S. D., Kerig, P. K., Bennett, D. C., & Modrowski, C. A. (2015). The roles of emotion dysregulation and dissociation in the association between sexual abuse and self-injury among juvenile justice-involved youth. *Journal of Trauma and Dissociation, 16*(3), 272–285. doi:10.1080/15299732.2015.989647

Charak, R., Byllesby, B. M., Roley, M. E., Claycomb, M. A., Durham, T. A., Ross, J., ... Elhai, J. D. (2016). Latent classes of childhood poly-victimization and associations with suicidal behavior among adult trauma victims: Moderating role of anger. *Child Abuse & Neglect, 62,* 19–28. doi:10.1016/j.chiabu.2016.10.010

Chartier, M. J., Walker, J. R., & Naimark, B. (2010). Separate and cumulative effects of adverse childhood experiences in predicting adult health and health care utilization. *Child Abuse & Neglect, 34*(6), 454–464. doi:10.1016/j.chiabu.2009.09.020

Cloitre, M., Stolbach, B. C., Herman, J. L., Van Der Kolk, B., Pynoos, R., Wang, J., & Petkova, E. (2009). A developmental approach to complex PTSD: Childhood and adult cumulative trauma as predictors of symptom complexity. *Journal of Traumatic Stress, 22*(5), 399–408. doi:10.1002/jts.20444

Collin-Vezina, D., & Hebert, M. (2005). Comparing dissociation and PTSD in sexually abused school-aged girls. *Journal of Nervous and Mental Disease, 193*(1), 47–52. 00005053-200501000-00008 [pii].

Cornelius, J. R., Kirisci, L., Reynolds, M., Clark, D. B., Hayes, J., & Tarter, R. (2010). PTSD contributes to teen and young adult cannabis use disorders. *Addictive Behavior, 35*(2), 91–94. S0306-4603(09)00236-6 [pii]. doi: 10.1016/j.addbeh.2009.09.007

Cudmore, R. M., Cuevas, C. A., & Sabina, C. (2015). The impact of polyvictimization on delinquency among Latino adolescents: A general strain theory perspective. *Journal of Interpersonal Violence.* doi:10.1177/0886260515593544

Cuevas, C. A., Finkelhor, D., Clifford, C., Ormrod, R. K., & Turner, H. A. (2010). Psychological distress as a risk factor for re-victimization in children. *Child Abuse and Neglect, 34*(4), 235–243. doi:10.1016/j.chiabu.2009.07.004

D'Andrea, W., Ford, J. D., Stolbach, B., Spinazzola, J., & Van Der Kolk, B. A. (2012). Understanding interpersonal trauma in children: Why we need a developmentally appropriate trauma diagnosis. *American Journal of Orthopsychiatry, 82*(2), 187–200. doi:10.1111/j.1939-0025.2012.01154.x

Danielson, C. K., Macdonald, A., Amstadter, A. B., Hanson, R., De Arellano, M. A., Saunders, B. E., & Kilpatrick, D. G. (2010). Risky behaviors and depression in conjunction with–Or in the absence of–Lifetime history of PTSD among sexually abused adolescents. [Research support, N.I.H., Extramural]. *Child Maltreatment, 15*(1), 101–107. doi:10.1177/1077559509350075

DeHart, D. D., & Moran, R. (2015). Poly-victimization among girls in the justice system: Trajectories of risk and associations to juvenile offending. *Violence Against Women, 21*(3), 291–312. doi:10.1177/1077801214568355

DePrince, A. P., Weinzierl, K. M., & Combs, M. D. (2008). Stroop performance, dissociation, and trauma exposure in a community sample of children. *Journal of Trauma and Dissociation, 9*(2), 209–223. doi:10.1080/15299730802048603

Dierkhising, C. B., & Branson, C. E. (2016). Looking forward: A research and policy agenda for creating trauma-informed juvenile justice systems. *Journal of Juvenile Justice, 5*(1), 14–30.

Dorahy, M. J. (2006). The dissociative processing style: Acognitive organization activated by perceived or actual threat in clinical dissociators. *Journal of Trauma and Dissociation, 7*(4), 29–53.

Dorahy, M. J., Corry, M., Shannon, M., Webb, K., McDermott, B., Ryan, M., & Dyer, K. F. (2013). Complex trauma and intimate relationships: The impact of shame, guilt and dissociation. *Journal of Affective Disorders, 147*(1–3), 72–79. doi:10.1016/j.jad.2012.10.010

Ehlers, C. L., Gizer, I. R., Gilder, D. A., Ellingson, J. M., & Yehuda, R. (2013). Measuring historical trauma in an American Indian community sample: Contributions of substance dependence, affective disorder, conduct disorder and PTSD. *Drug & Alcohol Dependence, 133*(1), 180–187. doi:10.1016/j.drugalcdep.2013.05.011

Estrada, A. L. (2009). Mexican Americans and historical trauma theory: A theoretical perspective. *Journal of Ethnicity and Subst Abuse, 8*(3), 330–340. doi:10.1080/15332640903110500

Finkelhor, D., Ormrod, R., Turner, H., & Holt, M. (2009). Pathways to poly-victimization. *Child Maltreatment, 14*(4), 316–329. 14/4/316 [pii]. doi: 10.1177/1077559509347012

Finkelhor, D., Ormrod, R. K., & Turner, H. A. (2007). Poly-victimization: A neglected component in child victimization. *Child Abuse & Neglect, 31*(1), 7–26. doi:10.1016/j.chiabu.2006.06.008

Finkelhor, D., Ormrod, R. K., & Turner, H. A. (2009). Lifetime assessment of poly-victimization in a national sample of children and youth. *Child Abuse & Neglect, 33*, 403–411. S0145-2134(09)00139-2 [pii]. doi:10.1016/j.chiabu.2008.09.012

Fite, P. J., Gabrielli, J., Cooley, J. L., Rubens, S. L., Pederson, C. A., & Vernberg, E. M. (2016). Associations between physical and relational forms of peer aggression and victimization and risk for substance use among elementary school-age youth. *Journal of Child & Adolescent Substance Abuse, 25*(1), 1–10. doi:10.1080/1067828X.2013.872589

Foote, B., Smolin, Y., Neft, D. I., & Lipschitz, D. (2008). Dissociative disorders and suicidality in psychiatric outpatients. *Journal of Nervous and Mental Disorders, 196*(1), 29–36. doi:10.1097/NMD.0b013e31815fa4e7

Ford, J. D. (2009). Dissociation in complex posttraumatic stress disorder or disorders of extreme stress not otherwise specified (DESNOS). In P. F. Dell, J. A. O'Neill, & E. Somer (Eds.), *Dissociation and the dissociative disorders: DSM-V and beyond* (pp. 471–485). New York, NY: Routledge.

Ford, J. D. (2017). Complex trauma and complex PTSD. In J. Cook, S. Gold, & C. Dalenberg (Eds.), *Handbook of trauma psychology* (Vol. 1, pp. 322–349). Washington, DC: American Psychological Association.

Ford, J. D., Chapman, J. C., Connor, D. F., & Cruise, K. R. (2012). Complex trauma and aggression in secure juvenile justice settings. *Criminal Justice & Behavior, 39*(5), 695–724.

Ford, J. D., Chapman, J., Mack, M., & Pearson, G. (2006). Pathways from traumatic child victimization to delinquency: Implications for juvenile and permanency court proceedings and decisions. *Juvenile and Family Court Journal, 57*(1), 13–26.

Ford, J. D., Connor, D. F., & Hawke, J. (2009). Complex trauma among psychiatrically impaired children: A cross-sectional, chart-review study. *Journal of Clinical Psychiatry, 70*(8), 1155–1163. doi:10.4088/JCP.08m04783

Ford, J. D., Elhai, J. D., Connor, D. F., & Frueh, B. C. (2010). Poly-victimization and risk of posttraumatic, depressive, and substance use disorders and involvement in delinquency in a national sample of adolescents. *Journal of Adolescent Health, 46*(6), 545–552. doi:10.1016/j.jadohealth.2009.11.212

Ford, J. D., Elhai, J. D., Ruggiero, K. J., & Frueh, B. C. (2009). Refining posttraumatic stress disorder diagnosis: Evaluation of symptom criteria with the national survey of adolescents. *Journal of Clinical Psychiatry, 70*(5), 748–755. doi:10.4088/JCP.08m04692

Ford, J. D., & Gomez, J. M. (2015). The relationship of psychological trauma and dissociative and posttraumatic stress disorders to nonsuicidal self-injury and suicidality: A review. *Journal of Trauma and Dissociation, 16*(3), 232–271. doi:10.1080/15299732.2015.989563

Ford, J. D., Grasso, D. J., Hawke, J., & Chapman, J. F. (2013). Poly-victimization among juvenile justice-involved youths. *Child Abuse and Neglect, 37*, 788–800. doi:10.1016/j.chiabu.2013.01.005

Ford, J. D., Hartman, J. K., Hawke, J., & Chapman, J. C. (2008). Traumatic victimization, posttraumatic stress disorder, suicidal ideation, and substance abuse risk among juvenile justice-involved youths. *Journal of Child and Adolescent Trauma, 1*, 75–92.

Ford, J. D., Kerig, P. K., Desai, N., & Feierman, J. (2016). Psychosocial interventions for traumatized youth in the juvenile justice system: Clinical, research, and legal perspectives. *Journal of Juvenile Justice, 5*(1), 31–49.

Ford, J. D., Wasser, T., & Connor, D. F. (2011). Identifying and determining the symptom severity associated with polyvictimization among psychiatrically impaired children in the outpatient setting. *Child Maltreatment, 16*(3), 216–226. 1077559511406109 [pii]. doi: 10.1177/1077559511406109

French, B. H., Bi, Y., Latimore, T. G., Klemp, H. R., & Butler, E. E. (2014). Sexual victimization using latent class analysis: Exploring patterns and psycho-behavioral correlates. *Journal of Interpersonal Violence, 29*(6), 1111–1131. doi:10.1177/0886260513506052

Gagnon, K. L., Lee, M. S., & DePrince, A. P. (2017). Victim-perpetrator dynamics through the lens of betrayal trauma theory. *Journal of Trauma and Dissociation,* 1–10. doi:10.1080/15299732.2017.1295421

Grasso, D., Greene, C., & Ford, J. D. (2013). Cumulative trauma in childhood. In J. D. Ford, & C. A. Courtois (Eds.), *Treating complex traumatic stress disorders in children and adolescents: An evidence based guide* (pp. 79–99). New York, NY: Guilford.

Grasso, D. J., Dierkhising, C. B., Branson, C. E., Ford, J. D., & Lee, R. (2015). Developmental patterns of adverse childhood experiences and current symptoms and impairment in youth referred for trauma-specific services. *Journal of Abnormal Child Psychology*. doi:10.1007/s10802-015-0086-8

Grisso, T., Barnum, R., Fletcher, K. E., Cauffman, E., & Peuschold, D. (2001). Massachusetts youth screening instrument for mental health needs of juvenile justice youths. *Journal of the American Academy of Child and Adolescent Psychiatry, 40*(5), 541–548. S0890-8567(09)60684-5 [pii]. doi: 10.1097/00004583-200105000-00013

Hamby, S., Finkelhor, D., & Turner, H. (2013). Perpetrator and victim gender patterns for 21 forms of youth victimization in the national survey of children's exposure to violence. *Violence and Victims, 28*(6), 915–939.

Jensen, S. A., Fabiano, G. A., Lopez-Williams, A., & Chacko, A. (2006). The reading grade level of common measures in child and adolescent clinical psychology. *Psychological Assessment, 18*(3), 346–352. doi:10.1037/1040-3590.18.3.346

Kelley, M. L., Klostermann, K., Doane, A. N., Mignone, T., Lam, W. K., Fals-Stewart, W., & Padilla, M. A. (2010). The case for examining and treating the combined effects of parental drug use and interparental violence on children in their homes. *Aggression and Violent Behavior, 15*(1), 76–82. doi:10.1016/j.avb.2009.09.002

Kerig, P. K., Bennett, D. C., Thompson, M., & Becker, S. P. (2012). "Nothing really matters": Emotional numbing as a link between trauma exposure and callousness in delinquent youth. *Journal of Traumatic Stress, 25*(3), 272–279. doi:10.1002/jts.21700

Kilic, O., Sar, V., Taycan, O., Aksoy-Poyraz, C., Erol, T. C., Tecer, O., … Ozmen, M. (2014). Dissociative depression among women with fibromyalgia or rheumatoid arthritis. *Journal of Trauma and Dissociation, 15*(3), 285–302. doi:10.1080/15299732.2013.844218

Kraemer, H. C. (2010). Epidemiological methods: About time. *International Journal of Environmetnal Research and Public Health, 7*(1), 29–45. doi:10.3390/ijerph7010029

Kuyken, W., & Dalgleish, T. (2011). Overgeneral autobiographical memory in adolescents at risk for depression. *Memory, 19*(3), 241–250. doi:10.1080/09658211.2011.554421

Lanius, R. A. (2015). Trauma-related dissociation and altered states of consciousness: A call for clinical, treatment, and neuroscience research. *European Journal of Psychotraumatology, 6*, 27905. doi:10.3402/ejpt.v6.27905

Lansing, A. E., Washburn, J. J., Abram, K. M., Thomas, U. C., Welty, L. J., & Teplin, L. A. (2014). Cognitive and academic functioning of juvenile detainees: Implications for correctional populations and public health. *Journal of Correctional Health Care, 20*(1), 18–30. doi:10.1177/1078345813505450

Le, M. T., Holton, S., Romero, L., & Fisher, J. (2016). Polyvictimization among children and adolescents in low- and lower-middle-income countries: A systematic review and meta-analysis. *Trauma, Violence & Abuse.* doi:10.1177/1524838016659489

Lee, M. A. (2015). Emotional abuse in childhood and suicidality: The mediating roles of re-victimization and depressive symptoms in adulthood. *Child Abuse and Neglect, 44*, 130–139. doi:10.1016/j.chiabu.2015.03.016

Leibowitz, G. S., Laser, J. A., & Burton, D. L. (2011). Exploring the relationships between dissociation, victimization, and juvenile sexual offending. *Journal of Trauma and Dissociation, 12*(1), 38–52. 932274936 [pii]. doi: 10.1080/15299732.2010.496143

Li, Y., Dong, F., Cao, F., Cui, N., Li, J., & Long, Z. (2013). Poly-victimization and executive functions in junior college students. *Scandinavian Journal of Psychology, 54*(6), 485–492. doi:10.1111/sjop.12083

Lucenko, B. A., Sharkova, I. V., Huber, A., Jemelka, R., & Mancuso, D. (2015). Childhood adversity and behavioral health outcomes for youth: An investigation using state administrative data. *Child Abuse and Neglect, 47*, 48–58. doi:10.1016/j.chiabu.2015.07.006

Mackinnon, D. P., Lockwood, C. M., & Williams, J. (2004). Confidence limits for the indirect effect: Distribution of the product and resampling methods. *Multivariate Behavioral Researcj, 39*(1), 99. doi: 10.1207/s15327906mbr3901_4

Maneta, E., Cohen, S., Schulz, M., & Waldinger, R. J. (2012). Links between childhood physical abuse and intimate partner aggression: The mediating role of anger expression. [Research support, N.I.H., extramural]. *Violence and Victims, 27*(3), 315–328.

McCullagh, C., Quinn, K., Voisin, D. R., & Schneider, J. (2017). A longitudinal examination of factors associated with social support satisfaction among HIV-positive young Black men who have sex with men. *AIDS Care*, 1–7. doi:10.1080/09540121.2017.1332333

McEwen, B., & Lasley, E. N. (2003). Allostatic load: When protection gives way to damage. *Advances in Mind-Body Medicine, 19*(1), 28–33.

McLaughlin, K. A. (2016). Future directions in childhood adversity and youth psychopathology. *Journal of Clinical Child and Adolescent Psychology, 45*(3), 361–382. doi:10.1080/15374416.2015.1110823

McLaughlin, K. A., Koenen, K. C., Hill, E. D., Petukhova, M., Sampson, N. A., Zaslavsky, A. M., & Kessler, R. C. (2013). Trauma exposure and posttraumatic stress disorder in a national sample of adolescents. *Journal of the American Academy of Child and Adolescent Psychiatry, 52*(8), 815–830 e814. doi:10.1016/j.jaac.2013.05.011

McLaughlin, K. A., & Sheridan, M. A. (2016). Beyond cumulative risk: A dimensional approach to childhood adversity. *Current Direrctions in Psychological Science, 25*(4), 239–245. doi:10.1177/0963721416655883

McReynolds, L. S., & Wasserman, G. A. (2011). Self-injury in incarcerated juvenile females: Contributions of mental health and traumatic experiences. *Journal of Traumatic Stress, 24* (6), 752–755. doi:10.1002/jts.20699

Messman-Moore, T. L., Walsh, K. L., & Dilillo, D. (2010). Emotion dysregulation and risky sexual behavior in revictimization. *Child Abuse and Neglect, 34*(12), 967–976. S0145-2134(10)00234-6 [pii]. doi: 10.1016/j.chiabu.2010.06.004

Miller-Graff, L. E., Cater, A. K., Howell, K. H., & Graham-Bermann, S. A. (2015). Victimization in childhood: General and specific associations with physical health problems in young adulthood. *Journal of Psychosomatic Research, 79*(4), 265–271. doi:10.1016/j.jpsychores.2015.07.001

Muthén, L. K., & Muthén, B. O. (2015). *Mplus user's guide (version 7.31)*. Los Angeles, CA: Muthén & Muthén.

Myhra, L. L. (2011). "It runs in the family": Intergenerational transmission of historical trauma among urban American Indians and Alaska natives in culturally specific sobriety maintenance programs. *American Indian and Alaska Native Mental Health Research, 18*(2), 17–40.

Olff, M., Polak, A. R., Witteveen, A. B., & Denys, D. (2014). Executive function in posttraumatic stress disorder (PTSD) and the influence of comorbid depression. *Neurobiology of Learning and Memory, 112*, 114–121. doi:10.1016/j.nlm.2014.01.003

Ouellet-Morin, I., Fisher, H. L., York-Smith, M., Fincham-Campbell, S., Moffitt, T. E., & Arseneault, L. (2015). Intimate partner violence and new-onset depression: A longitudinal study of women's childhood and adult histories of abuse. *Depression and Anxiety, 32*(5), 316–324. doi:10.1002/da.22347

Pereda, N., Abad, J., & Guilera, G. (2015). Victimization and polyvictimization of Spanish youth involved in juvenile justice. *Journal of Interpersonal Violence*. doi:10.1177/0886260515597440

Perron, B. E., Gotham, H. J., & Cho, D. (2008). Victimization among African-American adolescents in substance abuse treatment. *Journal of Psychoactive Drugs, 40*(1), 67–75.

Preacher, K. J., & Hayes, A. F. (2008). Asymptotic and resampling strategies for assessing and comparing indirect effects in multiple mediator models. *Behavior Research Methods, 40*(3), 879–891.

Radatz, D. L., & Wright, E. M. (2015). Does polyvictimization affect incarcerated and non-incarcerated adult women differently? An exploration into internalizing problems. *Journal of Interpersonal Violence.* doi:10.1177/0886260515588921

Ramiro, L. S., Madrid, B. J., & Brown, D. W. (2010). Adverse childhood experiences (ACE) and health-risk behaviors among adults in a developing country setting. *Child Abuse & Neglect, 34*(11), 842–855. doi:10.1016/j.chiabu.2010.02.012

Rauch, S. A., & Foa, E. B. (2006). Emotional processing theory (EPT) and exposure therapy for PTSD. [Electronic electronic; print]. *Journal of Contemporary Psychotherapy, 36*(2), 61–65.

Rivera-Velez, G. M., Gonzalez-Viruet, M., Martinez-Taboas, A., & Perez-Mojica, D. (2014). Post-traumatic stress disorder, dissociation, and neuropsychological performance in Latina victims of childhood sexual abuse. *Journal of Child Sexual Abuse, 23*(1), 55–73. doi:10.1080/10538712.2014.864746

Sar, V., Akyuz, G., Ozturk, E., & Alioglu, F. (2013). Dissociative depression among women in the community. *Journal of Trauma and Dissociation, 14*(4), 423–438. doi:10.1080/15299732.2012.753654

Scioli-Salter, E. R., Johnides, B. D., Mitchell, K. S., Smith, B. N., Resick, P. A., & Rasmusson, A. M. (2016). Depression and dissociation as predictors of physical health symptoms among female rape survivors with posttraumatic stress disorder. *Psychological Trauma, 8*(5), 585–591. doi:10.1037/tra0000135

Segura, A., Pereda, N., Guilera, G., & Abad, J. (2016). Poly-victimization and psychopathology among Spanish adolescents in residential care. *Child Abuse & Neglect, 55*, 40–51. doi:10.1016/j.chiabu.2016.03.009

Seng, J. S., D'Andrea, W., & Ford, J. D. (2014). Complex mental health sequelae of psychological trauma among women in prenatal care. *Psychological Trauma, 6*(1), 41–49. doi:10.1037/a0031467

Shane, P., Diamond, G. S., Mensinger, J. L., Shera, D., & Wintersteen, M. B. (2006). Impact of victimization on substance abuse treatment outcomes for adolescents in outpatient and residential substance abuse treatment. *American Journal on Addictions, 15*(Suppl 1), 34–42. L425802J7511H715 [pii]. doi: 10.1080/10550490601003714

Slopen, N., McLaughlin, K. A., Dunn, E. C., & Koenen, K. C. (2013). Childhood adversity and cell-mediated immunity in young adulthood: Does type and timing matter? *Brain, Behavior, and Immunity, 28*, 63–71. doi:10.1016/j.bbi.2012.10.018

Soler, L., Segura, A., Kirchner, T., & Forns, M. (2013). Polyvictimization and risk for suicidal phenomena in a community sample of Spanish adolescents. *Violence and Victimology, 28*(5), 899–912.

Southwick, S. M., Axelrod, S. R., Wang, S., Yehuda, R., Morgan, C. A., 3rd, Charney, D., … Mason, J. W. (2003). Twenty-four-hour urine cortisol in combat veterans with PTSD and comorbid borderline personality disorder. *The Journal of Nervous and Mental Disease, 191*(4), 261–262. doi:10.1097/01.NMD.0000061140.93952.28

Stansfeld, S. A., Clark, C., Smuk, M., Power, C., Davidson, T., & Rodgers, B. (2016). Childhood adversity and midlife suicidal ideation. *Psychological Medicine*, 1–14. doi:10.1017/S0033291716002336

Steinberg, A. M., Brymer, M. J., Kim, S., Briggs, E. C., Ippen, C. G., Ostrowski, S. A., … Pynoos, R. S. (2013). Psychometric properties of the UCLA PTSD reaction index: Part I. *Journal of Traumatic Stress, 26*(1), 1–9. doi:10.1002/jts.21780

Tamar-Gurol, D., Sar, V., Karadag, F., Evren, C., & Karagoz, M. (2008). Childhood emotional abuse, dissociation, and suicidality among patients with drug dependency in Turkey. *Psychiatry and Clinical Neurosciences, 62*(5), 540–547. doi:10.1111/j.1440-1819.2008.01847.x

Thompson, R., Flaherty, E. G., English, D. J., Litrownik, A. J., Dubowitz, H., Kotch, J. B., & Runyan, D. K. (2015). Trajectories of adverse childhood experiences and self-reported health at age 18. *Academic Pediatrics, 15*(5), 503–509. doi:10.1016/j.acap.2014.09.010

Turner, H. A., Finkelhor, D., & Ormrod, R. (2010). Poly-victimization in a national sample of children and youth. *American Journal of Preventive Medicine, 38*(3), 323–330. doi:10.1016/j.amepre.2009.11.012

Turner, H. A., Finkelhor, D., Shattuck, A., & Hamby, S. (2012). Recent victimization exposure and suicidal ideation in adolescents. *Archives of Pediatrics and Adolescent Medicine*, 1–6. doi:10.1001/archpediatrics.2012.1549

Turner, H. A., Shattuck, A., Finkelhor, D., & Hamby, S. (2016). Polyvictimization and youth violence exposure across contexts. *Journal of Adolescent Health, 58*(2), 208–214. doi:10.1016/j.jadohealth.2015.09.021

Van Dijke, A., Ford, J. D., Frank, L. E., & Van Der Hart, O. (2015). Association of childhood complex trauma and dissociation with complex posttraumatic stress disorder symptoms in adulthood. *Journal of Trauma and Dissociation, 16*(4), 428–441. doi:10.1080/15299732.2015.1016253

Voisin, D. R., Bird, J. D., Shiu, C. S., & Krieger, C. (2013). "It's crazy being a black, gay youth." Getting information about HIV prevention: A pilot study. *Journal of Adolescence, 36*(1), 111–119. doi:10.1016/j.adolescence.2012.09.009

Voisin, D. R., Hotton, A. L., Schneider, J. A., & Team, U. C. S. (2017). The relationship between life stressors and drug and sexual behaviors among a population-based sample of young Black men who have sex with men in Chicago. *AIDS Care, 29*(5), 545–551. doi:10.1080/09540121.2016.1224303

Wade, R., Jr., Cronholm, P. F., Fein, J. A., Forke, C. M., Davis, M. B., Harkins-Schwarz, M., … Bair-Merritt, M. H. (2016). Household and community-level adverse childhood experiences and adult health outcomes in a diverse urban population. *Child Abuse & Neglect, 52*, 135–145. doi:10.1016/j.chiabu.2015.11.021

Widom, C. S., Horan, J., & Brzustowicz, L. (2015). Childhood maltreatment predicts allostatic load in adulthood. *Child Abuse & Neglect, 47*, 59–69. doi:10.1016/j.chiabu.2015.01.016

4 Testing gender-differentiated models of the mechanisms linking polyvictimization and youth offending

Numbing and callousness versus dissociation and borderline traits

Patricia K. Kerig and Crosby A. Modrowski

ABSTRACT

The increasing prevalence of girls in the juvenile justice system suggests the importance of examining whether models of adolescent offending are differentiated by gender. Polyvictimization has emerged as a robust predictor of youth justice involvement, especially for girls, and research exploring mechanisms underlying the link between polyvictimization and offending suggests further gender differences in that callous-unemotional (CU) traits have been implicated in samples of boys whereas borderline personality (BP) traits have been implicated amongst girls. However, a limitation of these studies is that most have included all-male or all-female samples, thus not allowing for comparisons across gender. Further, few studies have used a trauma-informed lens to investigate posttraumatic symptoms, particularly dissociation and emotional numbing, that might account for these associations. To address this gap, this study investigated associations among polyvictimization, dissociation, numbing, CU, BP, and offending in a sample of 782 youth (579 boys and 203 girls) recruited from a detention center. As hypothesized, for both genders, polyvictimization was related to BP through the indirect effect of dissociation and to CU through the indirect effect of emotional numbing. Further, for both genders, path models indicated indirect effects on the association between polyvictimization and offending through dissociation and BP. These results suggest the value of using a trauma-informed approach to understanding youth justice involvement and continuing to fine-tune models of gender differences in traumatized girls' and boys' offending.

Recent decades have seen a striking increase in rates of arrest for juvenile offenses among adolescent girls. For example, the most recent decades have seen an 87% increase in girls' arrests for offenses against persons (Schwartz & Steffensmeier, 2012) and girls now account for 29 percent of juvenile arrests overall (Office of Juvenile Justice and Delinquency Prevention Databook, 2017). This dramatic increase in the "gender equity" of justice system involvement has highlighted the need to better understand the processes underlying girls' problem behavior (Kerig & Schindler, 2013; Zahn et al., 2010). A significant body of research confirms that key risks associated with youth justice involvement include posttraumatic stress symptoms, particularly those that arise in the context of polyvictimization (Ford, Elhai, Connor, & Frueh, 2010; Ford, Grasso, Hawke, & Chapman, 2013), which is defined as the experience of multiple forms of interpersonal victimization (Finkelhor, Ormrod, Turner, & Hamby, 2005). Moreover, victimization-related experiences and posttraumatic reactions have been shown in many studies to differentially predict problem behaviors among girls in comparison to boys (Burnette, Oshri, Lax, Richards, & Ragbeer, 2012; see Kerig & Becker, 2012). However, a number of questions remain unanswered concerning the underlying mechanisms accounting for the link between polyvictimization and delinquency; further, research has not yet explicated how polyvictimization and posttraumatic symptoms might be linked to other gender-linked sources of maladaptation associated with youth justice involvement, such as callous-unemotional (CU) and borderline personality (BP) traits. To contribute to our understanding of these issues, the present study examined gender differences in the associations among polyvictimization, posttraumatic symptoms, callous and borderline traits, and adolescent offending.

CU traits have emerged as significant predictors of adolescent entry into the justice system as well as the severity and recalcitrance of youth offenses (Frick, Ray, Thornton, & Kahn, 2014; Waller, Baskin-Sommers, & Hyde, 2017). However, much of this research has been based upon samples of boys and controversies have emerged regarding whether CU traits are equally relevant to girls' problem behavior. Measures of CU traits may not have the same predictive validity for girls (Colins, Damme, Andershed, Fanti, & DeLisi, 2017; Forouzan & Cooke, 2005), particularly in contrast to the stronger effects found for victimization-related variables within samples of female offenders (Odgers, Moretti, & Reppucci, 2009). For example, in a sample of detained girls, Odgers, Reppucci, and Moretti (2005) found that CU traits no longer contributed to the prediction of girls' aggression once maltreatment was entered into the equation. Moreover, research has called into question the assumption that CU traits emerge independently of trauma-related risk factors for delinquency. In several studies, adolescent CU traits have been found to be predicted by measures of childhood victimization, violence exposure, or maltreatment (Fontaine, McCrory, Boivin, Moffitt, & Viding, 2011; Kerig, Bennett, Thompson, & Becker, 2012; Kimonis, Fanti, Isoma, & Donoghue, 2013; Saukkonen et al., 2016; Sharf, Kimonis, & Howard, 2014; Waller, Baskin-Sommers, & Hyde, 2017; Waller, Gardner, & Hyde, 2013). Therefore, the current state of the field suggests the importance of examining CU traits and polyvictimization-linked risks in tandem, as well as investigating gender differences in their relative associations with justice involvement.

At the same time that some studies have questioned the utility of CU traits for understanding girls' justice involvement, other research has implicated a different trauma- and gender-linked dimension of adolescent personality, that of borderline personality (BP) traits. BP traits, including emotional, self, and interpersonal dysregulation, are associated with a history of childhood trauma and victimization (Hecht, Cicchetti, Rogosch, & Crick, 2014; Van Dijke, Ford, Van Son, Frank, & Van Der Hart, 2013) as well as with adolescent conduct problems (Beauchaine & McNulty, 2013; Chun et al., 2016), particularly for girls (Eppright, Kashani, Robison, & Reid, 1993). Furthermore, victimization predicts both BP and delinquent behavior in samples of adolescent girls (Penney & Lee, 2009). The value of BP for understanding girls' delinquency also is underscored by the finding that the association between childhood victimization and violent offending is mediated by the presence of BP in all-female samples (Burnette & Reppucci, 2009). However, an important limitation is that most studies of the link between BP traits and offending have included only girls and thus the presumption that BP is uniquely associated with girls' delinquency has not been tested. In two rare exceptions including boys, investigators have found that BP traits are also highly comorbid with boys' delinquent behaviors (Bradley, Conklin, & Westen, 2005) and that BP traits account for the association between victimization and offending for both genders (Chaplo, Kerig, Modrowski, & Bennett, 2017). Consequently, further research is needed to clarify whether BP traits are differentially associated with justice system involvement for girls in comparison to CU.

In addition, a new wave of work devoted to the role of victimization in youth justice involvement points to the importance of using a trauma-informed lens to better discern the underlying mechanisms that account for these associations (Ford & Blaustein, 2013; Ford et al., 2013; Kerig & Becker, 2010). For example, recent research regarding the link between victimization and CU traits has implicated the posttraumatic symptom of emotional numbing as a mechanism by which exposure to trauma comes to be expressed as callousness toward others and, consequently, results in delinquent behaviors (Allwood, Bell, & Horan, 2011; Kerig, Bennett et al., 2016). In a study testing this hypothesis in a detained sample including both genders, Kerig and colleagues (2012) found that posttraumatic emotional numbing statistically mediated the association between interpersonal trauma and CU traits. Therefore, the associations among polyvictimization, CU traits, and offending behaviors may be accounted for by the presence of posttraumatic emotional numbing. In turn, other trauma-informed research has implicated the posttraumatic symptom of dissociation as a mechanism underlying the BP traits demonstrated by traumatized male and female young offenders (Chaplo et al., 2017). Dissociation is prevalent among victimized boys and girls in the justice system (Bennett, Modrowski, Kerig, & Chaplo, 2015; Carrion & Steiner, 2000; Kerig, Charak et al., 2016) and is linked to BP both longitudinally (Zanarini, Frankenburg, Jager-Hyman, Reich, & Fitzmaurice, 2008) and cross-sectionally

(Chaplo, Kerig, Bennett, & Modrowski, 2015; Chaplo et al., 2017). Further, dissociation has been found to mediate the association between childhood victimization and BP in samples of maltreated boys and girls (Swannell et al., 2012).

In summary, given these suggestive findings, we hypothesized that, among polyvictimized adolescents in the juvenile justice system, posttraumatic numbing would be differentially related to CU traits whereas posttraumatic dissociation would be associated with BP traits and that, in turn, these trauma-related risks would account for gender differences in the association between polyvictimization and offending.

Method

Participants

Participants included 579 boys and 203 girls recruited from a short-term juvenile detention center in the western United States. Youth ranged in age from 12 to 19 years ($M = 16.07$, $SD = 1.30$) and, consistent with the ethnic composition of justice-involved youth in the geographic region from which they were drawn, 53.7% were White/Caucasian, 25.6% Hispanic/Latinx, 5.8% multi-racial, 3.8% Pacific Islander/Native Hawaiian, 5.1% Black/African American, 3.7% Native American/Alaskan Native, and 0.9% Asian American.

Measures

Polyvictimization
The UCLA Posttraumatic Stress Disorder Reaction Index for DSM-IV (PTSD-RI; Steinberg, Brymer, Decker, & Pynoos, 2004) is a widely-used screening tool which has demonstrated good convergent validity with other diagnostic measures, high internal consistency, and test-retest reliability over one week. The first set of questions asks youth whether they have been exposed to each of 13 specific traumatic events. The polyvictimization scale was comprised of a sum of six items involving victimization experiences (see Table 1) . Youth in the sample reported experiencing between 0 and 6 different forms of victimization ($M_{girls} = 2.72$, $SD = 1.58$; $M_{boys} = 2.53$, $SD = 1.38$) and the length of time elapsed since these events ranged from 3 to 180 months ($M = 33.19$, $SD = 37.30$).

Dissociation
The Adolescent Dissociative Experiences Scale (A-DES-II; Armstrong, Putnam, Carlson, Libero, & Smith, 1997) is a well-validated self-report measure designed to assess dimensions of dissociation (Kerig, Charak et al., 2016). Youth rate each item on an 11-point scale ranging from 0 (*never*) to 10 (*always*) and an average is calculated for each subscale. The score for the

Table 1. Victimization experiences reported by gender.

Victimization type	Girls		Boys		χ^2 (1, N = 782)
	n	%	n	%	
Family violence-witness	100	49.26	290	50.09	.07
Family violence-victim	58	28.57	166	28.67	.00
Sexual abuse	86	42.36	34	5.9	156.28***
Community violence-witness	136	67.00	386	66.67	.01
Community violence-victim	121	59.61	397	68.57	5.70*
Nonaccidental death/injury of loved one	110	54.19	284	49.05	1.75

*p < .05. *** p < .001.

depersonalization/derealization subscale (αs = 86 for girls, .87 for boys) was used in the present study, given that these are the symptoms used to define dissociation in the DSM-5 and research evidences these are the symptoms most indicative of pathological dissociation (Lanius et al., 2014).

Borderline traits

The Borderline Personality Features Scale (Crick, Murray-Close, & Woods, 2005) is a downward extension of the borderline scale on the Personality Assessment Inventory, including indices of affective instability, identity problems, negative relationships, and self-harm. Each of the 24 items is scored on a scale from 1 (*not at all true*) to 5 (*always true*). A total score summing all 24 items was used in the present analyses (αs = .86 for both genders).

Emotional numbing

The Emotional Numbing and Reactivity Scale (ENRS; Orsillo, Theodore-Oklota, Luterek, & Plumb, 2007) is a self-report assessing difficulty identifying and expressing feelings which has demonstrated reliability and validity in previous studies of adolescents (e.g., Allwood et al., 2011; Kerig, Bennett, Chaplo, Modrowski, & McGee, 2016). The general numbing subscale (8 items) was used in the present study. Item responses were rated on a five-point Likert-type scale ranging from 1 (*not at all typical of me*) to 5 (*very typical of me*) and were summed to create a total score (αs = .70 for girls, .71 for boys).

Callous-unemotional traits

The Inventory of Callous Unemotional Traits (ICU; (Kimonis et al., 2008) is a 24-item self-report measure that assesses lack of empathy and emotional responsiveness toward others. Each item is rated on a four-point Likert-style scale ranging from 1 = *not at all true* to 4 = *definitely true*. In keeping with recent recommendations (Ray, Frick, Thornton, Steinberg, & Cauffman, 2016), the total score was used in the present study (αs = .81 for girls, .76 for boys).

Offending behaviors

Self-reported delinquency was measured with a 33-item version of the Self Report of Delinquency (Elliott & Ageton, 1980), revised by Feiring, Miller-Johnson, and Cleland (2007) to include the low-level offenses that characterize girls in the justice system. Youth were asked to rate the number of times they had engaged in a variety of status offenses and illegal behaviors in the past year. The current study utilized a total score representing the number of times youth reported engaging in all events. The internal consistency of the measure in the current sample was good (αs = .93 for girls and boys).

Procedure

All study procedures were reviewed and approved by the Institutional Review Boards of the University of Utah and the Utah Department of Human Services. At visitations to detention centers, legal guardians provided signed informed consent, after which youth were invited to participate in the study. Youth who agreed provided signed assent, after which they completed study measures individually on a laptop computer in a private room within the detention center in the presence of a research assistant. Participants completed measures in the same order. No incentives were offered for participation. Data for the current study were collected between January 2011 and February 2014. Eighty eight percent of legal guardians who were approached agreed to participate in the study, whereas 71% of youth assented to participate.

Data analysis

Prior to conducting analyses, all variables were inspected for normality and outliers. Results of these inspections demonstrated that the offending variable had a skewed distribution (skewness = .82, SE = .16). We used structural equation modeling in M*plus* version 6.11 (Muthén & Muthén, 1998–2010) to examine direct and indirect effects among the variables. All variables were treated as observed and, given their association as reported in Table 2, dissociation and numbing were allowed to correlate. We utilized the robust maximum likelihood estimator (Brown, 2006). Adequacy of model fit was evaluated using root mean square error of approximation (RMSEA; Steiger, 1990), comparative fit index (CFI; Hu & Bentler, 1999), and root mean squared residual (SRMR). In order to investigate the possibility of moderation by gender, we utilized multigroup modeling in which factorial invariance was examined by comparing a constrained model in which all path coefficients were constrained to be equal for boys and girls to an unconstrained model using a chi square difference test.

Table 2. Descriptive statistics and gender differences.

Variable	Girls		Boys		
	Mean	SD	Mean	SD	t
Polyvictimization	2.72	1.58	2.35	1.38	3.19***
Dissociation	1.81	1.71	1.55	1.58	1.93*
Borderline traits	69.37	13.36	60.49	13.05	7.76***
Emotional numbing	17.32	5.53	17.35	5.07	−.09
Callous traits	27.04	9.17	27.10	8.24	−.08
Offending	73.77	28.85	74.23	31.18	−.10

*p < .05. *** p < .001.

Results

Descriptive statistics and main effects

Victimization experiences reported by youth in this sample are reported in Table 1. Comparisons of mean differences between boys and girls on all measures were performed using *t*-tests and are displayed in Table 2. Results indicated that girls reported higher levels of polyvictimization, BP, and dissociation in comparison to boys. Intercorrelations are shown separately by gender in Table 3.

Path model

Results indicated that the path model was a good fit to the data, RMSEA = .06, 90% CI = [.009, .131], CFI = .99, SRMR = .01. Tests for moderation by gender indicated that there was no significant difference between the models with constrained and unconstrained paths, $\chi2$ (13, $N = 782$) = 14.95, p = .31, suggesting invariance across gender. Figure 1 displays the path model testing the association between polyvictimization and offending and their indirect effects through dissociation and BP and through numbing and CU for the whole sample.

Table 3. Intercorrelations reported separately for girls and boys.

Variable	1.	2.	3.	4.	5.	6.
1. Polyvictimization	—	.31***	.27***	.28***	.17*	.44***
2. Dissociation	.14**	—	.48***	.50***	.19**	.24*
3. Borderline traits	.27***	.58***	—	.28***	.25***	.29*
4. Emotional numbing	.09*	.32***	.27***	—	.38***	.21
5. Callous traits	.08	.20***	.16**	.40***	—	.07
6. Offending	.36***	.20**	.36***	.20**	.13	—

Note. ns = 203 for girls and 579 for boys. Correlations for girls are displayed above the diagonal and correlations for boys are displayed in italics below the diagonal.
*p < .05. **p < .01. *** p < .001.

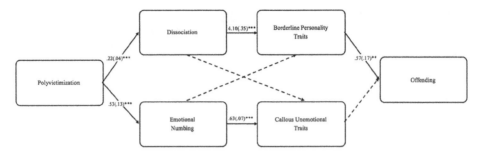

Figure 1. Path model for full sample. Only significant paths are displayed. Unstandardized coefficients (with standard errors in parentheses) are displayed for all significant paths. The direct effect from polyvictimization to offending is omitted from the figure for clarity but was included in the model. **$p < .01$. *** $p < .001$.

Direct effects

Results indicated a number of significant direct effects among the study variables. First, there was a significant direct effect between polyvictimization and offending, $B = 6.05$, $SE = 1.18$, $p < .001$. There also were significant associations between polyvictimization and emotional numbing, $B = .53$, $SE = .13$, $p < .001$, and polyvictimization and dissociation, $B = .22$, $SE = .04$, $p < .001$. Additionally, there were significant direct effects between BP and offending, $B = .57$, $SE = .17$, $p = .001$, numbing and CU, $B = .63$, $SE = .07$, $p < .001$, and BP and dissociation, $B = 4.1\text{-}$, $SE = .35$, $p < .001$.

Indirect effects

Results also suggested a number of indirect effects linking polyvictimization and offending. Specifically, results indicated that there was a significant indirect effect linking polyvictimization and BP through dissociation, $B = .89$, $SE = .18$, $p < .001$. Additionally, results demonstrated a significant indirect effect linking polyvictimization and CU through emotional numbing, $B = .33$, $SE = .09$, $p < .001$). Furthermore, there were significant indirect effects linking polyvictimization to offending through BP, $B = .98$, $SE = .33$, $p = .004$. Finally, results demonstrated a significant indirect effect linking polyvictimization and offending through both dissociation and BP traits, $B = .51$, $SE = .18$, $p = .005$.

Discussion

This study investigated gender similarities and differences in the associations among polyvictimization, trauma-linked symptoms, and offending in a sample of justice-involved adolescents. Specifically, we aimed to clarify whether there are gender-differentiated patterns in the risks for delinquency as has been suggested by studies implicating CU traits amongst boys versus BP traits amongst girls. Further, we sought to test the hypothesis that those traits were associated with specific posttraumatic symptoms. As expected, for both genders, polyvictimization was directly linked to offending; further, dissociation played an indirect role in the association between polyvictimization and BP traits whereas emotional numbing played an indirect role in the association between polyvictimization and CU traits.

Tests for overall gender differences in the study variables indicated findings consistent with other investigations of justice-involved youth, with girls reporting the highest rates of BP traits and dissociation, as well as the highest levels polyvictimization, particularly related to experiences of sexual abuse. In contrast, boys the highest levels of community violence. A well-replicated finding is that girls at risk or involved with delinquency report disproportionately more exposure to victimization in the context of close relationships, including maltreatment by parents and sexual abuse by dating partners (Cauffman, 2008; see Kerig & Schindler, 2013). Theory suggests that the betrayal accompanying these forms of intimate maltreatment may contribute to posttraumatic attempts to disavow the experience via dissociation (Chaplo et al., 2015; Freyd, 1996; Platt & Freyd, 2015) as well to the profound disruptions in self and interpersonal development that characterize BP traits (Chaplo et al., 2017; Kaehler & Freyd, 2012).

Next, we tested a model of the gender-differentiated associations among polyvictimization, posttraumatic symptoms, and offending. The results of path analyses suggested that, for both genders, dissociation had an indirect effect on the link between polyvictimization and BP. In turn, CU was linked indirectly to polyvictimization via emotional numbing for both genders. Unexpectedly, these indirect effects contributed to the prediction of offending only through the pathway of dissociation and BP and not through the pathway of CU and emotional numbing. These findings contrast with those of previous studies of the role of CU in offending and warrant further investigation and replication. However, although a cross-sectional study such as this cannot establish causality and must be interpreted with due caution, these results are consistent with the developmental psychopathology construct of equifinality, and suggest the possibility that posttraumatic symptoms involving affective, self, and interpersonal dysregulation may be particularly important to understanding the association between trauma and justice involvement. Further, these results suggest that research should continue to investigate CU traits through a trauma lens. In particular, attempts to understand the implications of CU among youth in the justice system should be informed by trauma-informed conceptualizations positing that, for some youth, CU may comprise not an inherent personality trait but rather an accommodation to a victimizing environment (Bennett & Kerig, 2014; Karpman, 1941; Porter, 1996).

Other investigations have indicated that BP might comprise a gender-linked risk for delinquency particular to girls (Burnette & Reppucci, 2009;

Penney & Lee, 2009) and, consistent with these prior studies, BP traits were directly linked to offending for girls here. However, in contrast to this proposed gender-specificity, polyvictimization-linked BP traits also were associated with offending for boys. As noted, this study is one of only a handful to include youth of both genders (Bradley et al., 2005; Chaplo et al., 2017), and the present results suggest that BP traits play an important if not well-recognized role in problem behavior amongst traumatized boys.

A number of limitations of this study are noteworthy. Although reports of polyvictimization were of events that occurred in the past, all variables were assessed cross-sectionally and thus the direction of effects cannot be established. Future research using longitudinal designs will be needed to test mediational hypotheses regarding the contributions of dissociation, BP, emotional numbing, and CU to our understanding of the polyvictimization-offending link. In addition, all variables were obtained via self-report and thus are subject to both mono-method and mono-informant biases. Moreover, polyvictimization was operationalized using a measure of traumatic experiences, which did not include other forms of victimization (e.g., bullying, property crimes) that are included in some scales. Further, this study followed a larger body of research in treating polyvictimization as a continuous variable (e.g., Cyr et al., 2013; Finkelhor et al., 2005). However, other investigations have typologized youth as polyvictims on the basis of cut-off scores, some of which, but not all, were higher than the mean number of victimization events found in the present sample (e.g., Ford et al., 2013). Using those alternative criteria would have truncated the current sample and may have yielded different results. Finally, these data were gathered in a detention center in a specific geographic region and may not be generalizable to a larger population.

Despite its limitations, the present study contributes to a growing body of literature devoted to understanding the ways in which childhood trauma exposure, particularly polyvictimization, contributes to the development of delinquent behavior in adolescence. These results suggest the value of using a trauma-informed approach to better elucidate the potential mechanisms underlying youth justice involvement and to increase our specificity regarding the posttraumatic symptoms that might disrupt adolescent functioning in ways that relate to justice system involvement. In addition, these findings speak to the importance of continuing to fine-tune our models related to gender differences in the effects of polyvictimization on girls' and boys' offending in order to better inform intervention efforts designed to deter at-risk youth from a delinquent pathway.

Acknowledgments

The authors wish to thank Anthony Fortuna for his valuable help with the preparation of this manuscript.

Disclosure statement

There are no conflicts of interest to report.

Funding

This work was funded by a grant from the National Institute of Justice (2014-90914-UT-IJ) to the first author and by a National Science Foundation Graduate Research Fellowship (No. 1256065) to the second author. Portions of an earlier version of this work were presented at the International Family Violence and Child Victimization Research Conference, Portsmouth, NH.

References

Allwood, M. A., Bell, D. J., & Horan, J. (2011). Posttrauma numbing of fear, detachment, and arousal predict delinquent behaviors in early adolescence. *Journal of Clinical Child and Adolescent Psychology, 40*(5), 659–667. doi:10.1080/15374416.2011.597081

Armstrong, J. G., Putnam, F. W., Carlson, E. B., Libero, D. Z., & Smith, S. R. (1997). Development and validation of a measure of adolescent dissociation: The Adolescent Dissociative Experiences Scale. *Journal of Nervous and Mental Disease, 185*(8), 491–497. doi:10.1097/00005053-199708000-00003

Beauchaine, T. P., & McNulty, T. (2013). Comorbidities and continuities as ontogenic processes: Toward a developmental spectrum model of externalizing psychopathology. *Development and Psychopathology, 25*(2), 1505–1528. doi:10.1017/S0954579413000746

Bennett, D. C., & Kerig, P. K. (2014). Investigating the construct of trauma-related acquired callousness among delinquent youth: Differences in emotion processing. *Journal of Traumatic Stress, 27*(4), 415–422. doi:10.1002/jts.21931

Bennett, D. C., Modrowski, C. A., Kerig, P. K., & Chaplo, S. D. (2015). Investigating the dissociative subtype of PTSD in a sample of traumatized detained youth. *Psychological Trauma, 7*(5), 465–472. doi:10.1037/tra0000057

Bradley, R., Conklin, C. Z., & Westen, D. (2005). The borderline personality diagnosis in adolescents: Gender differences and subtypes. *Journal of Child Psychology and Psychiatry, 46*(9), 1006–1019. doi:10.1111/j.1469-7610.2004.00401.x

Brown, T. A. (2006). *Confirmatory factor analysis for applied research.* New York, NY: Guilford Press.

Burnette, M. L., Oshri, A., Lax, R., Richards, D., & Ragbeer, S. N. (2012). Pathways from harsh parenting to adolescent antisocial behavior: A multidomain test of gender moderation. *Development and Psychopathology, 24*(3), 857–870. doi:10.1017/S0954579412000417

Burnette, M. L., & Reppucci, N. D. (2009). Childhood abuse and aggression in girls: The contribution of borderline personality disorder. *Development and Psychopathology, 21*(1), 309. doi:10.1017/S0954579409000170

Carrion, V. G., & Steiner, H. (2000). Trauma and dissociation in delinquent adolescents. *Journal of the American Academy of Child & Adolescent Psychiatry, 39*(3), 353–359. doi:10.1097/00004583-200003000-00018

Cauffman, E. (2008). Understanding the female offender. *Future of Children, 18*(2), 119–142. doi:10.1353/foc.0.0015

Chaplo, S. D., Kerig, P. K., Bennett, D. C., & Modrowski, C. A. (2015). The roles of emotion dysregulation and dissociation in the association between sexual abuse and self-injury among juvenile justice-involved youth. *Journal of Trauma & Dissociation, 16*(3), 272–285. doi:10.1080/15299732.2015.989647

Chaplo, S. D., Kerig, P. K., Modrowski, C. A., & Bennett, D. C. (2017). Gender differences in the sequelae of childhood sexual abuse: An examination of borderline features, dissociation, emotion dysregulation, and delinquent behaviors among detained adolescents. *Journal of Child and Adolescent Trauma, 10*(1). doi:10.1007/s40653-016-0122-z

Chun, S., Harris, A., Carrion, M., Rojas, E., Stark, S., Lejuez, C., ... Bornovalova, M. A. (2016). A psychometric investigation of gender differences and common processes across borderline and antisocial personality disorders. *Journal of Abnormal Psychology, 126*(1), 76–88. doi:10.1037/abn0000220

Colins, O. F., Damme, L., Andershed, H., Fanti, K. A., & DeLisi, M. (2017). Self-reported psychopathic traits and antisocial outcomes in detained girls. *Youth Violence and Juvenile Justice, 15*(2), 138–153. doi:10.1177/1541204015619659

Crick, N. R., Murray-Close, D., & Woods, K. (2005). Borderline personality features in childhood: A short-term longitudinal study. *Development and Psychopathology, 17*, 1051–1070. doi:10.1017/S0954579405050492

Cyr, K., Chamberland, C., Clement, M.-E., Lessard, G., Wemmers, J.-A., Collin-Vézina, D., ... Damant, D. (2013). Polyvictimization and victimization of children and youth: Results from a population survey. *Child Abuse & Neglect, 37*, 814–820. doi:10.1016/j.chiabu.2013.03.009

Elliott, D. S., & Ageton, S. S. (1980). Self-Reported Delinquency Questionnaire. *Psyctests.* doi:10.1037/t20796-000

Eppright, T., Kashani, J., Robison, B., & Reid, J. (1993). Comorbidity of conduct disorder and personality disorders in an incarcerated juvenile population. *American Journal of Psychiatry, 150*(8), 1233. doi:10.1176/ajp.150.8.1233

Feiring, C., Miller-Johnson, S., & Cleland, C. M. (2007). Potential pathways from stigmatization and internalizing symptoms to delinquency in sexually abused youth. *Child Maltreatment, 12*(3), 220–232. doi:10.1177/1077559507301840

Finkelhor, D., Ormrod, R., Turner, H., & Hamby, S. L. (2005). The victimization of children and youth: A comprehensive, national survey. *Child Maltreatment, 10*, 5–25. doi:10.1177/1077559504271287

Fontaine, N. M. G., McCrory, E. J. P., Boivin, M., Moffitt, T. E., & Viding, E. (2011). Predictors and outcomes of joint trajectories of callous–Unemotional traits and conduct problems in childhood. *Journal of Abnormal Psychology, 120*(3), 730–742. doi:10.1037/a0022620

Ford, J. D., & Blaustein, M. E. (2013). Systemic self-regulation: A framework for trauma-informed services in residential juvenile justice programs. *Journal of Family Violence, 28*, 665–677. doi:10.1007/s10896-013-9538-5

Ford, J. D., Elhai, J. D., Connor, D. F., & Frueh, B. C. (2010). Poly-victimization and risk of posttraumatic, depressive, and substance use disorders and involvement in delinquency in a national sample of adolescents. *Journal of Adolescent Health, 46*(6), 545–552. doi:10.1016/j.jadohealth.2009.11.212

Ford, J. D., Grasso, D. J., Hawke, J., & Chapman, J. F. (2013). Poly-victimization among juvenile justice-involved youths. *Child Abuse & Neglect, 37*(10), 788–800. doi:10.1016/j.chiabu.2013.01.005

Forouzan, E., & Cooke, D. J. (2005). Figuring out la femme fatale: Conceptual and assessment issues concerning psychopathy in females. *Behavioral Sciences & the Law, 23*(6), 765–778. doi:10.1002/bsl.669

Freyd, J. J. (1996). *Betrayal trauma: The logic of forgetting childhood abuse.* Cambridge: MA Harvard University Press.

Frick, P. J., Ray, J. V., Thornton, L. C., & Kahn, R. E. (2014). Annual research review: A developmental psychopathology approach to understanding callous-unemotional traits in children and adolescents with serious conduct problems. *Journal of Child Psychology and Psychiatry, 55*(6), 532–548. doi:10.1111/jcpp.12152

Hecht, K. F., Cicchetti, D., Rogosch, F. A., & Crick, N. R. (2014). Borderline personality features in childhood: The role of subtype, developmental timing, and chronicity of child maltreatment. *Development and Psychopathology, 26*(3), 805–815. doi:10.1017/S0954579414000406

Hu, L., & Bentler, P. M. (1999). Cutoff criteria for fit indexes in covariance structure analysis: conventional criteria versus new alternatives. *Structural Equation Modeling, 6,* 1–55. doi:10.1080/10705519909540118

Kaehler, L. A., & Freyd, J. J. (2012). Betrayal trauma and borderline personality characteristics: Gender differences. *Psychological Trauma, 4*(4), 379–385. doi:10.1037/a0024928

Karpman, B. (1941). On the need of separating psychopathy into two distinct clinical types: The symptomatic and the idiopathic. *Journal of Criminal Psychopathology, 3,* 112–137.

Kerig, P. K., & Becker, S. P. (2010). From internalizing to externalizing: Theoretical models of the processes linking PTSD to juvenile delinquency. In S. J. Egan (Ed.), *Posttraumatic stress disorder* (pp. 1–46). Hauppauge, NY: Nova Science Publishers.

Kerig, P. K., & Becker, S. P. (2012). Trauma and girls' delinquency. In S. Miller, L. D. Leve, & P. K. Kerig (Eds.), *Delinquent girls: Contexts, relationships, and adaptation* (pp. 119–143). New York, NY: Springer.

Kerig, P. K., Bennett, D. C., Chaplo, S. D., Modrowski, C. A., & McGee, A. B. (2016). Numbing of positive, negative, and general emotions: Associations with trauma exposure, posttraumatic stress, and depressive symptoms among justice-involved youth. *Journal of Traumatic Stress, 29*(2), 111–119. doi:10.1002/jts.22087

Kerig, P. K., Bennett, D. C., Thompson, M., & Becker, S. P. (2012). "Nothing really matters": Emotional numbing as a link between trauma exposure and callousness in delinquent youth. *Journal of Traumatic Stress, 25*(3), 272–279. doi:10.1002/jts.21700

Kerig, P. K., Charak, R., Chaplo, S. D., Bennett, D. C., Armour, C., Modrowski, C. A., & McGee, A. B. (2016). Validation of the factor structure of the adolescent dissociative experiences scale in a sample of trauma-exposed detained youth. *Psychological Trauma, 8* (5), 592–600. doi:10.1037/tra0000140

Kerig, P. K., & Schindler, S. R. (2013). Engendering the evidence base: A critical review of the conceptual and empirical foundations of gender-responsive interventions for girls' delinquency. *Laws, 2*(3), 244–282. doi:10.3390/laws2030244

Kimonis, E. R., Fanti, K. A., Isoma, Z., & Donoghue, K. (2013). Maltreatment profiles among incarcerated boys with callous-unemotional traits. *Child Maltreatment, 18*(2), 108–121. doi:10.1177/1077559513483002

Kimonis, E. R., Frick, P. J., Skeem, J. L., Marsee, M. A., Cruise, K., Munoz, L. C., ... Morris, A. S. (2008). Assessing callous-unemotional traits in adolescent offenders: Validation of the Inventory of Callous Unemotional traits. *International Journal of Law and Psychiatry, 31* (3), 241–252. doi:10.1016/j.ijlp.2008.04.002

Lanius, R. A., Wolf, E. J., Miller, M. W., Frewen, P. A., Vermetten, E., Brand, B., & Spiegel, D. (2014). The dissociative subtype of PTSD. In M. J. Friedman, T. M. Keane, & P. A. Resick (Eds.), *Handbook of PTSD* (2nd ed., pp. 234–250). New York, NY: Guilford.

Odgers, C. L., Moretti, M. M., & Reppucci, N. D. (2009). A review of findings from the "Gender and Aggression Project" informing juvenile justice policy and practice through gender-sensitive research. *Court Review, 46*(1–2), 6–8.

Odgers, C. L., Reppucci, N. D., & Moretti, M. M. (2005). Nipping psychopathy in the bud: An examination of the convergent, predictive, and theoretical utility of the PCL-YV among adolescent girls. *Behavioral Sciences & the Law, 23*(6), 743–763. doi:10.1002/bsl.664

Office of Juvenile Justice and Delinquency Prevention Databook. (2017). Retrieved October 10, 2017, from https://www.ojjdp.gov/ojstatbb/dmcdb

Orsillo, S. M., Theodore-Oklota, C., Luterek, J. A., & Plumb, J. (2007). The development and psychometric evaluation of the Emotional Reactivity and Numbing Scale. *Journal of Nervous and Mental Disease, 195*(10), 830–836. doi:10.1097/NMD.0b013e318156816f

Penney, S. R., & Lee, Z. (2009). Predicting and preventing aggression and violence risk in high-risk girls: Lessons learned and cautionary tales from the gender and aggression project. *Court Review, 46*(1–2), 36–43.

Platt, M. G., & Freyd, J. J. (2015). Betray my trust, shame on me: Shame, dissociation, fear, and betrayal trauma. *Psychological Trauma, 7*(4), 398–404. doi:10.1037/tra0000022

Porter, S. (1996). Without conscience or without active conscience? The etiology of psychopathy revisited. *Aggression and Violent Behavior, 1*(179-180). doi:10.1016/1359-1789(95)00010-0

Ray, J. V., Frick, P. J., Thornton, L. C., Steinberg, L., & Cauffman, E. (2016). Positive and negative item wording and its influence on the assessment of callous-unemotional traits. *Psychological Assessment, 28*(4), 394–404. doi:10.1037/pas0000183

Saukkonen, S., Aronen, E. T., Laajasalo, T., Salmi, V., Kivivuori, J., & Jokela, M. (2016). Victimization and psychopathic features in a population-based sample of Finnish adolescents. *Child Abuse & Neglect, 60*, 58–66. doi:10.1016/j.chiabu.2016.09.008

Schwartz, J., & Steffensmeier, D. (2012). Stability and change in girls' delinquency and the gender gap: Trends in violence and alcohol offending across multiple sources of evidence. In S. Miller, L. D. Leve, & P. K. Kerig (Eds.), *Delinquent girls: Context, relationships, and adaptation* (pp. 3–23). New York, NY: Springer.

Sharf, A., Kimonis, E. R., & Howard, A. (2014). Negative life events and posttraumatic stress disorder among incarcerated boys with callous-unemotional traits. *Journal of Psychopathology and Behavioral Assessment*, 1–14. doi:10.1007/s10862-013-9404-z

Steiger, J. H. (1990). Structural model evaluation and modification: An interval estimation approach. *Multivariate Behavioral Research, 25*, 173–180. doi: 10.1207/s15327906mbr2502_4

Steinberg, A. M., Brymer, M. J., Decker, K. B., & Pynoos, R. S. (2004). The University of California at Los Angeles Posttraumatic Stress Disorder Reaction Index. *Currrent Psychiatry Reports, 6*(2), 96–100. doi:10.1007/s11920-004-0048-2

Swannell, S., Martin, G., Page, A., Hasking, P., Hazell, P., Taylor, A., & Protani, M. (2012). Child maltreatment, subsequent non-suicidal self-injury and the mediating roles of dissociation, alexithymia and self-blame. *Child Abuse & Neglect, 36*, 572–584. doi:10.1016/j.chiabu.2012.05.005

Van Dijke, A., Ford, J. D., Van Son, M., Frank, L., & Van Der Hart, O. (2013). Association of childhood trauma by primary caregiver and affect dysregulation with borderline personality disorder symptoms in adulthood. *Psychological Trauma, 5*(3), 217–224. doi:10.1037/a0027256

Waller, R., Baskin-Sommers, A. R., & Hyde, L. W. (2017). Examining predictors of callous unemotional traits trajectories across adolescence among high-risk males. *Journal of Clinical Child & Adolescent Psychology.* doi:10.1080/15374416.2015.1102070

Waller, R., Gardner, F., & Hyde, L. W. (2013). What are the associations between parenting, callous-unemotional traits, and antisocial behavior in youth? A systematic review of evidence. *Clinical Psychology Review, 33*(4), 593–608. doi:10.1016/j.cpr.2013.03.001

Zahn, M. A., Agnew, R., Fishbein, D., Miller, S., Winn, D. M., Dakoff, G., ... Chesney-Lind, M. (2010). *Causes and correlates of girls' delinquency.* Washington, DC: Office of Juvenile Justice and Delinquency Prevention.

Zanarini, M. C., Frankenburg, F. R., Jager-Hyman, S., Reich, D. B., & Fitzmaurice, G. (2008). The course of dissociation for patients with borderline personality disorder and axis II comparison subjects: A 10-year follow-up study. *Acta Psychiatrica Scandinavica, 118*(4), 291–296. doi:10.1111/j.1600-0447.2008.01247.x

5   When stress becomes the new normal

Alterations in attention and autonomic
reactivity in repeated traumatization

Sarah Herzog 🄳, *Wendy D'Andrea, Jonathan DePierro,
and Vivian Khedari*

ABSTRACT
There is need for further work clarifying attention-physiology
interactions by degree of exposure to early victimization, as it
is clear that cumulative trauma in childhood, that is, polyvictimization, may have lasting effects on the stress response that
differ from those of acute traumatization. The present study
examined relationships between baseline and task-related physiology (indexed by respiratory sinus arrhythmia [RSA] and
heart rate [HR], respectively), and attention biases (via the
dot probe task), in 63 community-dwelling adult women stratified on the basis of self-reported exposure to multiple types
of childhood interpersonal victimization (i.e., sexual, physical,
and emotional abuse). Consistent with hypotheses, a pattern of
threat hypervigilance was found in the single victimization
group, while threat avoidance was found in the polyvictimization group. Additionally, avoidance of threat in the polyvictimized group was associated with lower baseline RSA.
Moderation analyses indicated that condition-wise HR moderated the relationship between level of exposure and attention
biases in the high-threat condition. The present findings may
clarify basic regulatory mechanisms that play a role in lifetime
revictimization in individuals with cumulative childhood
trauma exposure and may have implications for their prognostic and therapeutic outcomes.

After the experience of a traumatic event, such as a car accident, people may
avoid reminders of the trauma or experience intrusive memories about the
event. In such situations—post-traumatic stress disorder (PTSD) associated
with single-incident traumas—we find symptoms such as increased arousal
and hypervigilance for trauma reminders. But when the event is tragically
ordinary, occurring in multiple forms and setting, and across multiple years
of early life, the trauma is not isolated to a circumscribed set of reminders
one can avoid. We refer to the latter type of traumatization as complex

trauma, or polyvictimization (Courtois, 2008), and research suggests that trauma of this sort might be associated with a threat response that differs from the classic post-traumatic symptoms of hyperarousal and vigilance (D'Andrea, Pole, DePierro, Freed, & Wallace, 2013). Currently, however, alterations in threat responding in polyvictimized individuals remain little understood. The present study investigates differences in two central components of the threat response—attention and physiological reactivity—in adults with varying degrees of early lifetime trauma exposure.

Relative to acute trauma, polyvictimization requires a broader and more sustained adaptation to a cruel and inescapable reality (Cloitre et al., 2009; Van Der Kolk, Roth, Pelcovitz, Sunday, & Spinazzola, 2005). Complex childhood trauma is linked to alterations in physiological responses to stress or threat that persist into adulthood (Heim et al., 2000; Schmahl et al., 2004). For example, polyvictimization is related to enduring alterations in autonomic nervous system functioning following exposure (Van Der Kolk, 2002) that differ from the lasting autonomic effects associated with acute exposure (McTeague et al., 2010). Autonomic reactivity exerts significant influence on attention allocation (Gillie, Vasey, & Thayer, 2014; Thayer, Hansen, Saus-Rose, & Johnsen, 2009), and both autonomic and attentional processes are central elements of the threat response fundamental to basic survival (Bradley & Lang, 2000). Early life traumas are particularly likely to alter the threat response, since the brain undergoes significant growth during this period (Teicher, Andersen, Polcari, Anderson, & Navalta, 2002). Indeed, complex childhood trauma is known to have a lasting, pervasive impact on brain development (Teicher et al., 2004), cognitive functioning (Beers & De Bellis, 2002), and autonomic responding (Heim et al., 2000; Schmahl et al., 2004). Thus, the goal of this study is to investigate alterations in threat-related attention and autonomic reactivity in adults with histories of traumatic childhood victimization.

Alterations in attention allocation can take the form of selective attention toward threatening cues, an indication of hypervigilance (MacLeod, Mathews, & Tata, 1986), or bias away from threatening material, indicating avoidance (Koster, Crombez, Verschuere, & De Houwer, 2004; Price et al., 2012). These biases reflect both automatic, pre-attentive processes and more conscious strategies (Cisler & Koster, 2010). While both patterns of biased attention are associated with PTSD (Wald et al., 2011), patterns of threat avoidance might emerge as a byproduct of a dissociative adaptation to trauma, since dissociative processes function to reduce awareness of trauma-relevant information. An avoidant attentional bias might compromise processing of environmental dangers, thus conferring added risk of harm (Fani, Bradley-Davino, Ressler, & McClure-Tone, 2011). Clinically, rapid disengagement from trauma-related stimuli may also result in maintenance of symptoms by preventing consolidation of trauma memories (Foa, Steketee, & Rothbaum, 1989; Horowitz & Reidbord, 1992).

Attention bias findings in samples with childhood trauma histories are mixed; Gibb, Schofield, and Coles (2008) found that college students with histories of childhood maltreatment demonstrated hypervigilance for angry faces. In contrast, Pine et al. (2005) examined attention biases in maltreated children, all of whom had been exposed to severe domestic abuse. These researchers found that severity of physical abuse and a PTSD diagnosis were associated with bias away from threating faces. A growing number of studies have likewise linked PTSD symptom severity and trauma exposure in adults to attention biases away from threat (Elsesser, Sartory, & Tackenberg, 2004; Thomas, Goegan, Newman, Arndt, & Sears, 2013). However, at present, there is need for further research parsing the effects of accumulated types of abuse, more specifically childhood abuse, on attention biases.

Attention and cognitive control are reciprocally related to physiological activation of the autonomic nervous system (ANS), and both are regulated by similar brain systems (Thayer & Lane, 2000). Parasympathetic vagal activity, indexed through heart rate variability (HRV), is an indication of the degree to which the prefrontal cortex exerts inhibitory control over subcortical regions of the brain that extend to autonomic inputs in the heart, allowing the organism to respond flexibly and adaptively to environmental demands (Thayer & Lane, 2000). Studies have found lower HRV at rest in adults with PTSD compared to trauma-exposed individuals without PTSD, or controls (Cohen et al., 1998; Hauschildt, Peters, Moritz, & Jelinek, 2011; Sack, Hopper, & Lamprecht, 2004). Lower resting HRV, as indexed by respiratory sinus arrhythmia (RSA), was also associated with avoidance of anxiety-related words in women exposed to lifetime interpersonal violence (DePierro, D'Andrea, & Pole, 2013). Thus, HRV may be an important underlying factor in the flexibility of attention allocation.

Short-latency, or phasic, heart rate (HR) reactivity is thought to be a component of the attention-orienting response (Graham & Clifton, 1966) that is parasympathetically influenced, and responsive to threat intensity and proximity (Bradley et al, 2001). Growing evidence suggests that HR reactivity is not homogenous within traumatized samples. Soler-Baillo, Marx, and Sloan (2005) found decreased HR reactivity to auditory recordings of sexual coercion in adult sexual assault victims compared to non-traumatized controls. Conversely, higher HR reactivity to aversive stimuli has been found in a number of traumatized samples (for a review, see Orr, Metzger, and Pitman (2002)), including adults with histories of childhood trauma (Heim et al., 2000; Schmahl et al., 2004). Linking HR reactivity to attention, Elsesser et al. (2004) found that HR reactivity during a picture-viewing task in adults with chronic PTSD increased with the magnitude of attention bias toward trauma-related images. Additionally, attention directed away from trauma-related images was associated with greater intrusion symptoms. Patriquin, Wilson, Kelleher, and Scarpa (2012) found that sexually revictimized women demonstrated lower HR and parasympathetic activation at baseline and during an emotional Stroop task compared to those with childhood sexual assault only, despite no differences in reaction time to threatening and trauma-related words. Thus, autonomic threat reactivity varies across traumatized samples, and these differences may be accounted for by unique patterns of traumatization across the lifetime.

In summary, while both altered attentional and autonomic threat reactivity are associated with trauma exposure and symptoms, research has yet to investigate whether attention and physiology shift as a function of the degree of trauma exposure during the sensitive developmental period of early life. Accordingly, the present study aimed to investigate relations between early interpersonal victimization and threat-related attention biases and the potential moderating role of autonomic reactivity. We operationalized victimization as acts of commission (e.g., actual or threatened abuse of any kind) and did not include acts of omission (e.g., neglect) in accordance with prior work (Cuevas, Sabina, & Picard, 2010; Widom, Czaja, & Dutton, 2008). Polyvictimization was operationalized as exposure to multiple domains of abuse. Along with trauma exposure, trauma-related symptoms that might plausibly impact attention were also assessed. We hypothesized that directionality of threat-related bias would change as a function of accumulated trauma exposure, such that greater traumatization would be associated with a bias away from threat, as suggested in the literature (Elsesser et al., 2004; Pine et al., 2005; Thomas et al., 2013), and lower-level victimization associated with bias toward threat. Attenuated baseline HRV was expected to be associated with avoidance of threat at higher levels of victimization, and hypervigilance at lower levels of victimization. Finally, avoidance of threat in polyvictimized individuals was expected to be associated with greater HR reactivity to threat trials. As an ancillary hypothesis, trauma-related symptoms were expected to differentially impact patterns of attention, such that non-dissociative PTSD symptoms would be related to vigilance, while dissociative symptoms would be related to threat avoidance.

Method

Participants

Seventy-five female participants were recruited from the NYC area using online advertisements. Inclusion criteria required participants be between ages 18 to 55 and comfortable reading and writing in English. The sample had a mean age of 33.10 (SD = 10.01) and was diverse with respect to race/ethnicity; over 70% of the overall sample represented non-white minority members, with 36.5% identifying as African American/Black, and 20% as Hispanic/Latino (see Table S1 in *Supplemental Materials*).

Approximately 70% of participants ($n = 44$) reported at least one category of childhood victimization (i.e., physical, sexual, or emotional abuse), 46% ($n = 29$) reported physical abuse, 38% ($n = 24$) reported sexual abuse, and 52.4% ($n = 33$) reported emotional abuse. Of the sample, 30% ($n = 19$) did not endorse any of the above categories of IPV in childhood. While childhood emotional and physical neglect were not included in IPV analyses, 70% of the sample endorsed the former, and 49% the latter.

Measures and materials

Traumatic events screening inventory-brief report form (TESI-BR)

Lifetime trauma was assessed on the TESI-BR, a 12-item scale assessing exposure to potentially traumatic events such as natural disasters, illness, accidents, injuries, violence, and sexual assault (Ford & Fournier, 2007). This scale was used to compute the earliest age of trauma exposure, as well as an index of interpersonal traumas (sexual, physical, and emotional) occurring before age 16.

Childhood trauma questionnaire (CTQ)

The CTQ is a 28-item self-report measure for exposure to childhood abuse and neglect, assessing severity of exposure across five domains: emotional abuse, physical abuse, sexual abuse, emotional neglect, and physical neglect (Bernstein & Fink, 1998).

Multiscale dissociation inventory (MDI; Briere, 2002)

The MDI is a 30-item self-report measure used to assess dissociative symptomatology in the past month. The frequency of occurrence of each item is rated on a 5-point scale (1 = "never", 5 = "very often"). The measure provides a total severity score, as well as six subscales: disengagement, depersonalization, derealization, memory disturbance, emotional constriction, and identity dissociation. Internal consistency for the full scale was high, $a = .95$.

PTSD checklist for DSM 5 (PCL-5; Weathers et al., 2013)

The PCL-5, a self-report measure of PTSD symptoms occurring in the past month, contains 20 symptoms that comprise DSM-5 criteria B through E (i.e., intrusions, avoidance, negative alterations in cognitions and mood, and alterations and arousal and reactivity symptom clusters). Symptom severity over the past month is rated on a 5-point scale (0 = "not at all", 5 = "extremely"). Internal consistency for total score was high, $a = .95$.

Visual dot-probe task

Fifty pictures from the International Affective Picture System (Lang, Bradley, & Cuthbert, 1999) were selected according to normative ratings for valence and arousal, including five highly threatening images (e.g., "mutilated face"), five mildly threatening images (e.g., "man with knife"), five positive images (e.g., "couple laughing"), and thirty-five neutral pictures (e.g., "hair dryer"). See Table S2 in *Supplementary Materials* for normed arousal and valence ratings by condition and Table S3 for a listing of stimuli.

Heart rate

HR is a measure of the chronotropic activity of the heart, which is controlled by innervation from the sympathetic (SNS) and parasympathetic (PNS) nervous systems (Andreassi, 2007). Participants were instructed on how to place three Mindware ECG sensors (Mindware Technologies Ltd., Gahanna, OH) on their chests in Lead II configuration (one below the right clavicle, one below the right ribcage, and one below the left ribcage). ECG signal was sampled at 1000 Hz using BioLab software (MindWare Technologies, Gahanna, OH). HR was calculated offline using custom software (HRV3.0; MindWare Technologies, Gahanna, OH).

Respiratory sinus arrhythmia (RSA)

RSA indexes PNS activity and is a well-validated measure of HRV. RSA was derived through spectral analysis of the high-frequency band (0.12–0.40 Hz) of the inter-beat interval, using Mindware Software (HRV3.0; MindWare Technologies, Gahanna, Ohio).

Procedure

An Institutional Review Board approved the present study. All procedures took place within a university laboratory setting. After providing informed consent, participants completed self-report measures, had sensors affixed to measure physiology, and underwent a two-minute resting baseline from which HR and RSA were derived. Participants were administered the dot-probe task, during which concurrent HR was measured. Upon completion, participants were compensated $25.

The dot-probe task was implemented in E-Prime 2.0 (Psychology Software Tools, Pittsburgh, PA) and included 16 practice trials and 100 randomly sequenced experimental trials consisting of 40 neutral, 20 high-threat, 20 mild-threat, and 20 positive trials. Trials began with presentation of a fixation cross for 500 ms, followed by a pair of images presented side by side for 1000 ms, consistent with time frames used to study complex images (Miller & Fillmore, 2010). Presentation of the paired images was immediately replaced by a probe either in the position of the emotional image (congruent trials) or in the position of the neutral image (incongruent trials), for a duration of 1000 ms. For each trial type, probe position was alternated to create congruent (i.e., probe in experimental position) and incongruent trials (probe in neutral position), and images were alternated on each side of the screen, resulting in 20 trials per experimental condition (5 images × 2 probe position × 2 image position). Participants were directed to respond with keypresses as quickly as possible to the position of the probe on the screen.

Data preparation and analysis

Dot-probe data preparation

Bias toward threat is indicated when reaction times (RT) are shorter for congruent trials than incongruent trials (Koster et al., 2004). Thus, a negative difference score in RT indicates bias away from valenced stimuli, and a positive score indicates a bias toward valenced stimuli. The resulting formula was as follows: Bias = Mean Incongruent Trial RT - Mean Congruent Trial RT. Bias scores were computed for high-threat condition, mild-threat conditions, and positive conditions.

Behavioral data reduction

Of 75 total cases, three with missing dot-probe data (due to software malfunction or participant aborting the protocol prematurely) and four with fewer than 10 valid trials were excluded from analysis. Following standard practice, trials with RTs <100 ms (Mogg, Mathews, & Eysenck, 1992), "lapses" (trial RTs >1000 ms), and "errors" (i.e., incorrect responses) were eliminated; thereafter, participants whose excluded trials exceeded 10% of total trials were removed from the final analyses. Five participants were thus eliminated, leaving a total of 63 participants. Excluded and included participants did not significantly differ with respect to age, minority status (i.e., white versus non-white), sexual orientation, socioeconomic status, symptoms, and baseline physiology.

Physiological data preparation

Physiological data was visually inspected for quality using software that flags unusual variations in inter-beat intervals as possible artifacts created by movement (Mindware HRV 3.0; Mindware Inc, Gahanna: OH). Using this guideline, noise was removed for approximately half of all participants. HR was parsed in trial-wise sequences, resulting in 100 segments of ~2 s epochs. Trial-wise HR data was averaged within stimulus conditions to provide condition-wise HR reactivity for high-threat, mild-threat, neutral, and positive stimuli. Trial-wise data was missing for two participants, one of whom was removed due to excessive artifacts. Baseline physiological data was missing for one participant.

A note on physiological data interpretation

HR increases with sympathetic activation and decreases with parasympathetic (i.e., vagal), activation; conversely, HR decreases with sympathetic withdrawal and increases with parasympathetic withdrawal. Because of this, HR measured over long periods of time cannot be used to infer the differential influence of SNS versus PNS activity on chronotropic changes. However, short-term chronotropic demands allow for interpretation of whether HR fluctuations are due to SNS or PNS activity. Specifically, SNS inputs cannot influence HR in fewer than 3 s, whereas PNS activity can produce changes in HR within 1 s. Thus, chronotropic changes occurring within each 2 s trial of the dot probe task are more likely attributable to PNS changes, wherein higher HR may be related to vagal withdrawal, and lower HR related to vagal activation. However, since it can be difficult to determine whether physiology during a given trial represents a discrete reaction to that trial rather than accumulated carryover effects from the stressful stimuli preceding it, interpretation should be made with caution.

Data analysis

To perform tests of moderation, we used PROCESS (Model 1; Hayes, 2015), an add-on macro for SPSS that implements moderation and mediation analysis using a path analysis framework (Hayes, 2012). PROCESS also quantifies direct and indirect effects using bias-corrected bootstrapped samples of 1,000, and conditional effects for moderation analyses. General linear modeling and all other analyses were performed in SPSS.

Results

Classification of victimization

To provide a categorical measure of interpersonal victimization (IPV), endorsement of commission traumas (e.g., physical, sexual, and emotional abuse) on either the TESI (before age 16) or CTQ were used to create dichotomous groups based on trauma type. Then, polyvictimization groups were created based on endorsement of either one, two, or three of the aforementioned categories of IPV.

Of the overall sample, 24% ($n = 15$) endorsed only one abuse category, hereon referred to as single traumatization (e.g., Type 1 IPV). Sixteen participants (25.4%) endorsed two categories (e.g., Type 2), and 20.6% ($n = 13$) reported three categories of abuse, that is., polyvictimization (or Type 3). Participants who did not endorse any IPV were included in continuous analyses only and are presented alongside IPV groups in Table 1 and S1 for comparison purposes.

Table 1. Physiological and attention scores by polyvictimization group.

		No Child IPV*	Type 1 IPV	Type 2 IPV	Type 3 IPV
Baseline Physiology	HR	75.27 (9.58)	73.35 (8.74)	71.35 (11.60)	73.06 (13.12)
	RSA	6.01 (1.37)	6.24 (1.15)	6.56 (1.04)	6.11 (1.27)
	Condition				
Task-Related	HT	76.00 (11.86)	75.48 (75.06)	74.28 (13.34)	74.55 (13.93)
Heart Rate	MT	75.21 (11.18)	75.59 (10.03)	74.57 (13.50)	75.39 (14.23)
	Neutral	75.24 (11.27)	75.82 (9.23)	74.42 (13.22)	74.67 (14.78)
	Positive	75.77 (11.13)	75.01 (8.82)	75.07 (12.82)	74.13 (14.02)
Reaction Time	HT	592.37 (157.18)	548.68 (128.41)	536.74 (124.85)	652.46 (240.46)
	MT	573.35 (131.44)	532.08 (115.82)	535.01 (125.86)	614.98 (165.21)
	Neutral	560.37 (135.45)	523.77 (119.07)	519.74 (116.71)	597.19 (174.89)
	Positive	564.89 (136.03)	528.09 (127.63)	515.94 (117.14)	588.70 (151.66)
Attention Bias	HT	−4.92 (48.68)	27.45 (56.06)	18.30 (60.88)	−26.02 (56.05)
	MT	11.64 (49.26)	−14.23 (53.23)	8.07 (62.38)	15.43 (93.49)
	Positive	−23.92 (74.68)	−17.18 (60.19)	3.72 (62.19)	−30.89 (57.66)

Abbreviations: IPV = interpersonal victimization, HR = heart rate, RSA = respiratory sinus arrhythmia, HT = high-threat, MT = mild-threat
Note: IPV groups (Types 1, 2, and 3) are based on endorsement of either 1, 2, or 3 categories of childhood IPV. All values reflect mean scores.
*Not included in group-wise IPV analyses.

Race/ethnicity (white vs. non-white) and age did not differ between those with and without IPV, or across IPV group. Dissociative and PTSD symptoms did not differ by IPV group. Childhood physical and emotional neglect did significantly differ by IPV group; post-hoc pairwise comparisons indicated that the polyvictimized group had significantly higher emotional neglect scores than the singly victimized group. No other pairwise comparisons of neglect were significant.

Dot-probe data

Table 1 provides descriptive data of the reaction time and attention bias scores in each dot-probe condition (i.e., high-threat, mild threat, etc.), presented by IPV group.

Attention bias and polyvictimization

One-way ANOVAs tested the effects of IPV group status on attention biases in each condition. Attention biases in the high-threat condition differed by polyvictimization group ($F[2,41] = 3.35$, $p = .045$, $M_{diff} = 39.46$, $d = 0.75$). Post-hoc pairwise comparisons indicated significant differences in between Type 1 and Type 3 groups, with the latter group (i.e., polyvictimized) demonstrating bias away from threat, and the former demonstrating bias toward threat. Groups did not differ in bias to mild-threat or positive conditions.

Table 2. Bivariate correlations for self-report and behavioral measures.

Variables	1	2	3	4	5	6	7	8	9	10	11	12
1. CTQ Total												
2. PCL-5 Total	.49**											
3. MDI Total	.44**	.74**										
4. Age of Trauma Onset	−.32*	−.28*	−.27*									
5. Baseline HR	−.08	−.04	−.27*	.15								
6. Baseline RSA	.04	.08	.26*	−.20	−.58**							
7. HT RT	.05	.24	.10	−.12	.16	−.27*						
8. MT RT	.03	.18	.03	−.08	.16	−.31*	.95**					
9. Neutral RT	.05	.22	.11	−.10	.11	−.29*	.96**	.97**				
10. Positive RT	.02	.20	.05	−.11	.12	−.29*	.95**	.95**	.98**			
11. HT Bias	−.15	.01	.01	−.17	−.12	.04	.13	.13	.12	.19		
12. MT Bias	.23	.31*	.08	.16	.17	−.30*	.48**	.43**	.50**	.46**	.11	
13. Positive Bias	.04	.19	.17	.04	−.06	.06	−.00	−.01	−.01	−.01	.18	.18

Abbreviations: CTQ = Childhood Trauma Questionnaire, PCL-5 = PTSD Checklist for DSM 5, MDI = Multiscale Dissociation Inventory, HR = heart rate, RSA = respiratory sinus arrhythmia, HT = high-threat, MT = mild-threat, RT = reaction time.
*Correlation is significant at the 0.05 level (2-tailed). **Correlation is significant at the 0.01 level (2-tailed).

Physiological data

Table 1 provides descriptive data for baseline heart rate and RSA, and heart rate in each dot-probe condition, presented by IPV group. Baseline HR and RSA did not differ by IPV group. Baseline RSA correlated negatively with bias scores in the mild-threat condition, suggesting that hypervigilance is associated with lower RSA (see Table 2 for correlations).

Attention bias and physiology

Baseline RSA was plotted against bias scores in the high-threat condition and stratified by group. Type 1 and Type 2 groups demonstrated a bias toward threat at lower baseline RSA values (see Figure 1). Inversely, in the Type 3 group, lower RSA values were associated with bias away from threat, and higher values were associated with bias toward threat. In the mild-threat condition (see Figure 2), all three groups demonstrated bias toward threat at lower levels of RSA. A multivariate ANCOVA on threat bias scores by group, with baseline RSA entered as a covariate, demonstrated a significant main effect for group ($F(3,74) = 2.77$, $p = .033$, $\eta^2 = .13$). There was no main effect for RSA ($F(1,36) = 2.18$, $p = .127$, $\eta^2 = .11$), and a marginally significant RSA × group interaction ($F(3,74) = 2.10$, $p = .090$, $\eta^2 = .10$). For high-threat bias, there was a significant between-subjects effect for group ($F(2,37) = 4.90$, $p = .013$, $\eta^2 = .21$), and group × RSA ($F(2,37) = 3.81$, $p = .031$, $\eta^2 = .17$). Pairwise comparisons indicated an avoidant pattern in the high-threat condition for the Type 3 group ($M = -22.69$, $SE = 15.44$) that significantly differed from the hypervigilant scores of Type 1 ($M = 26.54$, $SE = 14.28$, $M_{diff} = -49.22$, $p = .025$) and Type 2 ($M = 26.90$, $SE = 14.73$, $M_{diff} = -49.59$, $p = .026$) groups. For mild-threat bias, there was a significant between-

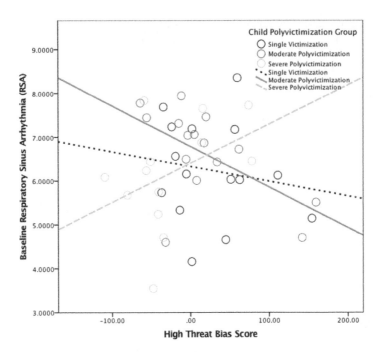

Figure 1. Relationship between baseline Respiratory Sinus Arrhythmia (RSA) and high-threat bias by polyvictimization group.

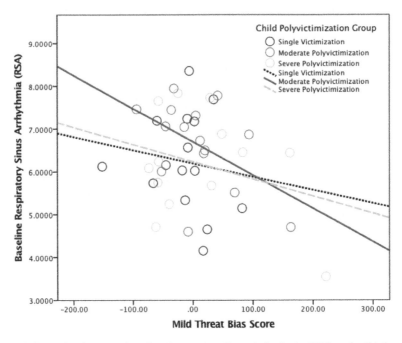

Figure 2. Relationship between baseline Respiratory Sinus Arrhythmia (RSA) and mild-threat bias by polyvictimization group.

Table 3. Moderating effect of condition-wise mean HR on relationship between child polyvictimization and bias scores.

Models	B (SE)	t	p	R^2	F
Model 1: High-Threat	–	–	.015	.237	3.94
Constant	−116.53 (113.19)	−1.03	.31	–	–
Child Polyvictimization	140.85 (80.15)	1.76	.087	–	–
Mean HR High-Threat Trials	1.99 (1.49)	1.33	.190	–	–
Group × HR	−2.25 (1.06)	−2.13	.040	.091	4.52
Model 2: Mild-Threat	–	–	.612	.046	0.61
Constant	23.19 (123.83)	0.19	.852	–	–
Child Polyvictimization	−47.33 (90.74)	−0.52	.605	–	–
Mean HR Mild-Threat Trials	−0.43 (1.63)	−0.26	.794	–	–
Group × HR	0.81 (1.18)	0.69	.497	.012	0.47
Model 3: Positive	–	–	.541	.054	0.73
Constant	142.61 (121.19)	1.18	.246	–	–
Child Polyvictimization	−120.50 (85.58)	−1.41	.167	–	–
Mean HR Positive Trials	−2.00 (1.60)	−1.25	.219	–	–
Group × HR	1.52 (1.13)	1.34	.189	.045	1.79

Abbreviations: HR = heart rate.

subjects effect for RSA ($F(1,37) = 4.22$, $p = .047$, $\eta^2 = .10$), but no significant difference in bias scores across IPV groups.

To investigate the contribution of HR reactivity to attention biases, moderation analyses were conducted for each condition (see Table 3). Bias scores per condition were entered as the dependent variable, polyvictimization groups entered as the predictor variable, and the corresponding condition-wise mean HR entered as the moderating variable. For the high-threat condition, the overall model was significant and accounted for approximately 24% of the variance in high-threat bias, $p = .015$. Polyvictimization was marginally significant in the model, $p = .087$. Mean HR for high-threat trials did not significantly contribute to the model, either, $p = .190$. However, the interaction between condition-wise HR × polyvictimization was significant, $p = .040$, R^2-change $= .091$, such that those in the severe polyvictimization group with higher HR in the high-threat condition demonstrated avoidance of threat (see Figure 3). A Johnson-Neyman test of significance regions demonstrated that HR values at or above 72.779 (approximately the 52nd percentile) significantly influenced the relationship between polyvictimization and avoidance of threat.

The moderation model was replicated for the mild-threat and positive conditions. There were no significant main effects for either model (see Table 3).

Self-reported symptoms

Total PTSD symptoms correlated positively with mild-threat bias, indicating that symptom severity increased with hypervigilance. Although total dissociative symptoms were not significantly related to bias scores, the

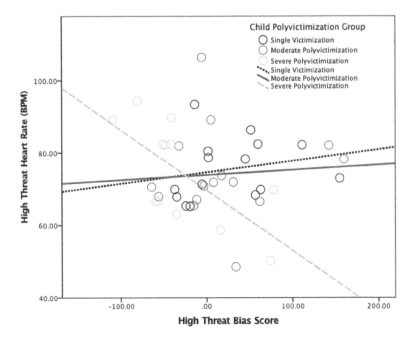

Figure 3. Interaction between high-threat condition HR (in beats per minute) and polyvictimization group on high-threat bias.

dissociative depersonalization subscale was significantly associated with bias toward threat in the mild-threat condition. Because dissociative and PTSD symptoms were highly intercorrelated in this sample ($r = .74$), posthoc partial correlations were conducted, controlling for PTSD symptoms (see Table S5 in *Supplemental Materials*). Total dissociative symptoms were marginally negatively correlated with mild-threat bias. Subscales of dissociative disengagement, emotion constriction, and memory disturbance were significantly negatively correlated with mild-threat bias, indicating avoidance of threat.

Discussion

The current study examined attention biases to threat and concurrent physiological responding in community-sampled adults. Consistent with stated hypotheses, threat-related attention biases in the high-threat condition differed as a function of the extent of trauma exposure, such that individuals reporting a single category of victimization (Type 1) demonstrated hypervigilance, whereas those with polyvictimization (Type 3) demonstrated an avoidant pattern. Results support the main hypothesis that attention biases may emerge as a result of accumulated trauma exposure in early life. Much like the current sample, differing profiles of attention biases across traumatized samples have been found in a number of previous studies. Thomas et al. (2013) found that time-course patterns of attention differed as a function of PTSD symptoms severity, wherein participants with sub-threshold symptoms demonstrated sustained, heightened attention to threatening images, while more severe PTSD symptoms were related to initial hypervigilance, followed by avoidance. Reichert, Segal, and Flannery-Schroeder (2015) investigated differences in attention biases across levels of repeated traumatization in a sample of college students and did not find group-wise differences; however, this study examined interpersonal and non-interpersonal traumas alike and did not differentiate between traumas occurring in childhood and those later in life.

Patterns of attention biases in this study also differed as a function of degree of stimulus threat: mild-threat was associated with hypervigilance, and the high-threat condition was associated with avoidance. This pattern has been similarly evinced in previous research; Bryant and Harvey (1997), for example, found participants with PTSD demonstrated hypervigilance to mildly threatening stimuli but no bias toward high-threat stimuli. In the current sample, PTSD symptoms were likewise associated with bias to mild-threat, while no associations were demonstrated in the high-threat condition. Thus, it is possible that hypervigilant threat responses are more visible in the context of benign threat cues, or "hints" at danger, so to speak, whereas obvious danger may be more likely to provoke avoidance.

The current study built upon the existing literature by assessing baseline autonomic physiology, and concurrent cardiovascular reactivity to dot-probe trials, with the expectation that amplified sympathetic responses to threat would be related to alterations in attention, specifically avoidance. Indeed, our findings demonstrated an interaction between HR responses on the high-threat trials, and attention biases on such trials, wherein amplified HR moderated the relationship between greater trauma exposure and avoidance of threat. Thus, an avoidant response to threatening stimuli might reflect an effort to down-regulate anxiety-related bodily cues such as dysregulated cardiovascular responses (i.e., increased HR). This interpretation is consistent with theoretical work linking disinhibition of the autonomic nervous system in anxiety disorders to behavioral avoidance (Friedman & Thayer, 1998). Since the chronotropic effects of the parasympathetic system are deployed more rapidly than sympathetic stimulation, it is also possible that trial-wise HR changes indexed in the current sample are a product of variation in parasympathetic control, rather than sympathetic reactivity.

Results were consistent with our hypothesis that attention bias would be differentially related to baseline vagal tone across polyvictimization groups. Low vagal tone at baseline was associated with attentional avoidance in those with greater polyvictimization (Type 3), whereas for lower levels of victimization, dampened baseline vagal tone was associated with bias toward threat, or hypervigilance. In the overall sample, which includes both victimized and non-victimized individuals, baseline RSA was negatively correlated with threat bias in the mild-threat condition, indicating that bias toward threat may be more pronounced at lower levels of RSA. Additionally, in the polyvictimized group, an HR of approximately 73 bpm predicted a bias away from threat, a value within the normal range of resting human HR (Palatini, 1999). This suggests a low tolerance for physiological arousal in this group, wherein even slight reactivity to aversive stimuli is associated with an avoidant response. Thus, for highly victimized clients, tolerating negative affect and increasing capacity for self-regulation, as indexed by high RSA, may be a treatment goal that differentiates polyvictimized from singly victimized individuals. Indeed, preliminary research demonstrates that HRV biofeedback effectively increases HRV while reducing PTSD symptoms (Zucker, Samuelson, Muench, Greenberg, & Gevirtz, 2009).

Attention biases may also be differentially impacted by trauma-related symptoms. In the current sample, DSM-5 PTSD symptoms were associated with hypervigilance, while dissociative symptoms were associated with avoidance. The common links between polyvictimization, dissociation, and threat avoidance mirror the existing literature; in instances of complex or chronic trauma in early childhood, it is not uncommon for a persistent tendency to dissociate in threatening contexts to emerge over time (Howell, 2013). The tendency to dissociate under stress, however, might have the adverse effect of slowing processing of threat-related cues (Kluft, 1990), making trauma survivors more vulnerable to continued exposure to potentially traumatic events (Sandberg, Matorin, & Lynn, 1999).

Limitations

The present study is limited by a number of factors. First, measures of trauma history and symptoms were assessed via self-report, rather than in-person interviews. Additionally, due to the cross-sectional study design, we are unable to state definitively whether alterations in attention are due to trauma incurred in childhood, or if they preceded the trauma. It also remains possible that attention biases are influenced by traumas occurring in adulthood. Moreover, without the supplement of eye tracking, we are unable to state without doubt whether longer latencies in response to threat represent avoidance of attention or slowed psychomotor responses.

In the current study, stimulus presentation duration was supraliminal, that is, 1000 ms, long enough to be consciously perceived. It could be argued that longer latencies obscure measurement of the automatic orienting response, which involve earlier (<500 ms) preconscious processes (Mathews & MacLeod, 1986). However, a number of previous dot-probe studies have found evidence of vigilance using longer latencies ($\geq$ 1000 ms) of exposure

(Bradley, Mogg, White, Groom, & Bono, 1999; Dalgleish et al., 2003; Naim et al., 2014). For example, Mogg, Bradley, De Bono, and Painter (1997) found vigilance toward threat across exposures of 100, 500, and 1500 ms, with no significant differences between durations. Thus, it is likely that both pre-attentive processes and more conscious strategies play a role in attention bias (Cisler & Koster, 2010).

Implications

While PTSD-related studies commonly index a single reference trauma, many individuals experience multiple traumas of varying types by the time they reach adulthood, with multiple traumas being the norm (Briere, Kaltman, & Green, 2008). In the current study, cumulative childhood trauma was related to attentional avoidance of threating images, and concurrent autonomic reactivity to threat. Research on the impact of early-life polyvicti-mization on core regulatory capacities (i.e., attention and autonomic reactiv-ity) might provide important insights into the specific needs of individuals with complex trauma and inform clinical interventions adjusted to their unique symptom profile. More broadly, however, such work would allow us to extend beyond hypervigilance models of PTSD to better account for the heterogeneity in trauma-related symptoms, attention biases, and treatment outcomes.

Funding

This study was funded by the 2014 International Society for the Study of Trauma and Dissociation David Caul Research Grant.

ORCID

Sarah Herzog ⓘ http://orcid.org/0000-0001-9161-3061

References

Andreassi, J. (2007). Heart activity and behavior. II. Stress, emotions, motivation, personality, social factors, brain interactions, and conditioning. *Psychophysiology: Human Behavior and Physiological Response*. Hillsdale, NJ: Lawrence Erlbaum.

Beers, S. R., & De Bellis, M. D. (2002). Neuropsychological function in children with maltreatment-related posttraumatic stress disorder. *American Journal of Psychiatry, 159* (3), 483–486. doi:10.1176/appi.ajp.159.3.483

Bernstein, D. P., & Fink, L. (1998). *Childhood trauma questionnaire: A retrospective self-report:*. Manual. San Antonio, TX: The Psychological Corporation.

Bradley, M. M., Codispoti, M., Cuthbert, B. N., & Lang, P. J. (2001). Emotion and motivation I: defensive and appetitive reactions in picture processing. *Emotion, 1*(3), 276.

Bradley, B. P., Mogg, K., White, J., Groom, C., & Bono, J. (1999). Attentional bias for emotional faces in generalized anxiety disorder. *British Journal of Clinical Psychology, 38* (3), 267–278. doi:10.1348/014466599162845

Bradley, M. M., & Lang, P. J. (2000). Measuring emotion: Behavior, feeling, and physiology. *Cognitive Neuroscience of Emotion, 25,* 49–59.

Briere, J. (2002). *MDI, Multiscale dissociation inventory: Professional manual.* Odessa, FL: Psychological Assessment Resources.

Briere, J., Kaltman, S., & Green, B. L. (2008). Accumulated childhood trauma and symptom complexity. *Journal of Traumatic Stress, 21*(2), 223–226. doi:10.1002/(ISSN)1573-6598

Bryant, R. A., & Harvey, A. G. (1997). Attentional bias in posttraumatic stress disorder. *Journal of Traumatic Stress, 10*(4), 635–644. doi:10.1002/jts.2490100409

Cisler, J. M., & Koster, E. H. (2010). Mechanisms of attentional biases towards threat in anxiety disorders: An integrative review. *Clinical Psychology Review, 30*(2), 203–216. doi:10.1016/j.cpr.2009.11.003

Cloitre, M., Stolbach, B. C., Herman, J. L., Kolk, B. V. D., Pynoos, R., Wang, J., & Petkova, E. (2009). A developmental approach to complex PTSD: Childhood and adult cumulative trauma as predictors of symptom complexity. *Journal of Traumatic Stress, 22*(5), 399–408. doi:10.1002/jts.20444

Cohen, H., Kotler, M., Matar, M. A., Kaplan, Z., Loewenthal, U., Miodownik, H., & Cassuto, Y. (1998). Analysis of heart rate variability in posttraumatic stress disorder patients in response to a trauma-related reminder. *Biological Psychiatry, 44*(10), 1054–1059. doi:10.1016/S0006-3223(97)00475-7

Courtois, C. A. (2008). Complex trauma, complex reactions: Assessment and treatment. *Psychological Trauma: Theory, Research, Practice, and Policy,* (1), 86–100.

Cuevas, C. A., Sabina, C., & Picard, E. H. (2010). Interpersonal victimization patterns and psychopathology among Latino women: Results from the SALAS study. *Psychological Trauma: Theory, Research, Practice, and Policy, 2*(4), 296. doi:10.1037/a0020099

D'Andrea, W., Pole, N., DePierro, J., Freed, S., & Wallace, D. B. (2013). Heterogeneity of defensive responses after exposure to trauma: Blunted autonomic reactivity in response to startling sounds. *International Journal of Psychophysiology, 90*(1), 80–89. doi:10.1016/j.ijpsycho.2013.07.008

Dalgleish, T., Taghavi, R., Neshat-Doost, H., Moradi, A., Canterbury, R., & Yule, W. (2003). Patterns of processing bias for emotional information across clinical disorders: A comparison of attention, memory, and prospective cognition in children and adolescents with depression, generalized anxiety, and posttraumatic stress disorder. *Journal of Clinical Child and Adolescent Psychology, 32*(1), 10–21. doi:10.1207/S15374424JCCP3201_02

DePierro, J., D'Andrea, W., & Pole, N. (2013). Attention biases in female survivors of chronic interpersonal violence: relationship to trauma-related symptoms and physiology. *European Journal of Psychotraumatology, 4*(0). doi:10.3402/ejpt.v4i0.19135

Elsesser, K., Sartory, G., & Tackenberg, A. (2004). Attention, heart rate, and startle response during exposure to trauma-relevant pictures: A comparison of recent trauma victims and patients with posttraumatic stress disorder. *Journal of Abnormal Psychology, 113*(2), 289–301. doi:10.1037/0021-843x.113.2.289

Fani, N., Bradley-Davino, B., Ressler, K. J., & McClure-Tone, E. B. (2011). Attention bias in adult survivors of childhood maltreatment with and without posttraumatic stress disorder. *Cognitive Therapy and Research, 35*(1), 57–67. doi:10.1007/s10608-010-9294-2

Foa, E. B., Steketee, G., & Rothbaum, B. O. (1989). Behavioral/cognitive conceptualizations of post-traumatic stress disorder. *Behavior Therapy, 20*(2), 155–176. doi:10.1016/S0005-7894 (89)80067-X

Ford, J. D., & Fournier, D. (2007). Psychological trauma and post-traumatic stress disorder among women in community mental health aftercare following psychiatric intensive care. *Jpi*, *3*(01). doi:10.1017/s1742646407001094

Friedman, B. H., & Thayer, J. F. (1998). Autonomic balance revisited: Panic anxiety and heart rate variability. *Journal of Psychosomatic Research*, *44*(1), 133–151. doi:10.1016/S0022-3999 (97)00202-X

Gibb, B. E., Schofield, C. A., & Coles, M. E. (2008). Reported history of childhood abuse and young adults' information processing biases for facial displays of emotion. *Child Maltreatment*, *14*(2), 148–156.

Gillie, B. L., Vasey, M. W., & Thayer, J. F. (2014). Heart rate variability predicts control over memory retrieval. *Psychological Science*, *25*(2), 458–465. doi:10.1177/0956797613508789

Graham, F. K., & Clifton, R. K. (1966). Heart-rate change as acomponent of the orienting response. *Psychological bulletin*, *65*(5), 305.

Hauschildt, M., Peters, M. J., Moritz, S., & Jelinek, L. (2011). Heart rate variability in response to affective scenes in posttraumatic stress disorder. *Biological Psychology*, *88*(2), 215–222. doi:10.1016/j.biopsycho.2011.08.004

Hayes, A. F. (2015). *Hacking PROCESS to Estimate a Simple Moderation Model With a Three Category Moderator*. Unpublished white paper, Department of Psychology, The Ohio State University, Columbus, OH.

Hayes, A. F. (2012). *PROCESS: A versatile computational tool for observed variable mediation, moderation, and conditional process modeling. [White paper]*. Retrieved from http://www. afhayes.com/public/process2012.pdf

Heim, C., Newport, D. J., Heit, S., Graham, Y. P., Wilcox, M., Bonsall, R., . . . Nemeroff, C. B. (2000). Pituitary-adrenal and autonomic responses to stress in women after sexual and physical abuse in childhood. *Jama*, *284*(5), 592–597. doi:10.1001/jama.284.5.592

Horowitz, M. J., & Reidbord, S. P. (1992). Memory, emotion, and response to trauma. In S.-Å. Christianson (Ed.), *The Handbook of Emotion and Memory: Research and Theory* (pp. 343–357). Hillsdale, NJ: Lawrence Erlbaum Associates, Inc.

Howell, E. F. (2013). *The dissociative mind* (pp. 25). New York, NY: Routledge.

Kluft, R. P. (1990). Dissociation and subsequent vulnerability: A preliminary study. *Dissociation: Progress in the Dissociative Disorders*, *3*(3), 167–173.

Koster, E. H. W., Crombez, G., Verschuere, B., & De Houwer, J. (2004). Selective attention to threat in the dot probe paradigm: Differentiating vigilance and difficulty to disengage. *Behaviour Research and Therapy*, *42*(10), 1183–1192. doi:10.1016/j.brat.2003.08.001

Lang, P. J., Bradley, M. M., & Cuthbert, B. N. (1999). International affective picture system (IAPS): Instruction manual and affective ratings. *The center for research in psychophysiology*, University of Florida.

MacLeod, C., Mathews, A., & Tata, P. (1986). Attentional bias in emotional disorders. *Journal of Abnormal Psychology*, *95*(1), 15–20. doi:10.1037/0021-843x.95.1.15

Mathews, A., & MacLeod, C. (1986). Discrimination of threat cues without awareness in anxiety states. *Journal of Abnormal Psychology*, *95*(2), 131. doi:10.1037/0021-843X.95.2.131

McTeague, L. M., Lang, P. J., Laplante, M.-C., Cuthbert, B. N., Shumen, J. R., & Bradley, M. M. (2010). Aversive imagery in posttraumatic stress disorder: Trauma recurrence, comorbidity, and physiological reactivity. *Biological Psychiatry*, *67*(4), 346–356. doi:10.1016/j. biopsych.2009.08.023

Miller, M. A., & Fillmore, M. T. (2010). The effect of image complexity on attentional bias towards alcohol-related images in adult drinkers. *Addiction*, *105*(5), 883–890. doi:10.1111/ j.1360-0443.2009.02860.x

Mogg, K., Bradley, B. P., De Bono, J., & Painter, M. (1997). Time course of attentional bias for threat information in non-clinical anxiety. *Behaviour Research and Therapy*, *35*(4), 297–303. doi:10.1016/S0005-7967(96)00109-X

Mogg, K., Mathews, A., & Eysenck, M. (1992). Attentional bias to threat in clinical anxiety states. *Cognition & Emotion*, *6*(2), 149–159. doi:10.1080/02699939208411064

Naim, R., Wald, I., Lior, A., Pine, D., Fox, N. A., Sheppes, G., ... Bar-Haim, Y. (2014). Perturbed threat monitoring following a traumatic event predicts risk for post-traumatic stress disorder. *Psychological Medicine*, *44*(10), 2077–2084. doi:10.1017/S0033291713002456

Orr, S. P., Metzger, L. J., & Pitman, R. K. (2002). Psychophysiology of post-traumatic stress disorder. *Psychiatric Clinics*, *25*(2), 271–293.

Palatini, P. (1999). Need for a revision of the normal limits of resting heart rate. *Hypertension*, *33*(2), 622–625. doi:10.1161/01.HYP.33.2.622

Patriquin, M. A., Wilson, L. C., Kelleher, S. A., & Scarpa, A. (2012). Psychophysiological reactivity to abuse-related stimuli in sexually revictimized women. *Journal of Aggression, Maltreatment & Trauma*, *21*(7), 758–775. doi:10.1080/10926771.2012.690835

Pine, D. S., Mogg, K., Bradley, B. P., Montgomery, L., Monk, C. S., McClure, E., ... Kaufman, J. (2005). Attention bias to threat in maltreated children: Implications for vulnerability to stress-related psychopathology. *American Journal of Psychiatry*, *162*(2), 291–296. doi:10.1176/appi.ajp.162.2.291

Price, R. B., Siegle, G. J., Silk, J. S., Ladouceur, C., McFarland, A., Dahl, R. E., & Ryan, N. D. (2012). Sustained neural alterations in anxious youth performing an attentional bias task: A pupilometry study. *Depression and Anxiety*, *30*(1), 22–30. doi:10.1002/da.21966

Reichert, E., Segal, C., & Flannery-Schroeder, E. (2015). Trauma, attentional biases, and revictimization among young adults. *Journal of Trauma & Dissociation*, *16*(2), 181–196. doi:10.1080/15299732.2014.975308

Sack, M., Hopper, J. W., & Lamprecht, F. (2004). Low respiratory sinus arrhythmia and prolonged psychophysiological arousal in posttraumatic stress disorder: Heart rate dynamics and individual differences in arousal regulation. *Biological Psychiatry*, *55*(3), 284–290. doi:10.1016/S0006-3223(03)00677-2

Sandberg, D. A., Matorin, A. I., & Lynn, S. J. (1999). Dissociation, posttraumatic symptomatology, and sexual revictimization: A prospective examination of mediator and moderator effects. *Journal of Traumatic Stress*, *12*(1), 127–138. doi:10.1023/a:1024702501224

Schmahl, C. G., Elzinga, B. M., Ebner, U. W., Simms, T., Sanislow, C., Vermetten, E., ... Bremner, J. D. (2004). Psychophysiological reactivity to traumatic and abandonment scripts in borderline personality and posttraumatic stress disorders: A preliminary report. *Psychiatry Research*, *126*(1), 33–42. doi:10.1016/j.psychres.2004.01.005

Soler-Baillo, J. M., Marx, B. P., & Sloan, D. M. (2005). The psychophysiological correlates of risk recognition among victims and non-victims of sexual assault. *Behav Res Ther*, *43*(2), 169–181. doi:10.1016/j.brat.2004.01.004

Teicher, M. H., Andersen, S. L., Polcari, A., Anderson, C. M., & Navalta, C. P. (2002). Developmental neurobiology of childhood stress and trauma. *Psychiatric Clinics*, *25*(2), 397–426.

Teicher, M. H., Dumont, N. L., Ito, Y., Vaituzis, C., Giedd, J. N., & Andersen, S. L. (2004). Childhood neglect is associated with reduced corpus callosum area. *Biological Psychiatry*, *56*(2), 80–85. doi:10.1016/j.biopsych.2004.03.016

Thayer, J. F., Hansen, A. L., Saus-Rose, E., & Johnsen, B. H. (2009). Heart rate variability, prefrontal neural function, and cognitive performance: The neurovisceral integration perspective on self-regulation, adaptation, and health. *Annals of Behavioral Medicine*, *37*(2), 141–153. doi:10.1007/s12160-009-9101-z

Thayer, J. F., & Lane, R. D. (2000). A model of neurovisceral integration in emotion regulation and dysregulation. *Journal of Affective Disorders, 61*(3), 201–216. doi:10.1016/S0165-0327(00)00338-4

Thomas, C. L., Goegan, L. D., Newman, K. R., Arndt, J. E., & Sears, C. R. (2013). Attention to threat images in individuals with clinical and subthreshold symptoms of post-traumatic stress disorder. *Journal of Anxiety Disorders, 27*(5), 447–455. doi:10.1016/j.janxdis.2013.05.005

Van Der Kolk, B. A. (2002). The assessment and treatment of complex PTSD. In R. Yehuda (Ed.), *Treating Trauma Survivors with PTSD* (pp. 127–156). Washington, DC: American Psychiatric Publishing, Inc.

Van Der Kolk, B. A., Roth, S., Pelcovitz, D., Sunday, S., & Spinazzola, J. (2005). Disorders of extreme stress: The empirical foundation of a complex adaptation to trauma. *Journal of Traumatic Stress, 18*(5), 389–399. doi:10.1002/(ISSN)1573-6598

Wald, I., Shechner, T., Bitton, S., Holoshitz, Y., Charney, D. S., Muller, D., ... Bar-Haim, Y. (2011). Attention bias away from threat during life threatening danger predicts PTSD symptoms at one-year follow-up. *Depression and Anxiety, 28*(5), 406–411. doi:10.1002/da.20808

Weathers, F., Litz, B., Keane, T., Palmieri, P., Marx, B., & Schnurr, P. (2013). *The PTSD checklist for DSM-5 (PCL-5)*. Scale available at from the National Center for PTSD at http://www.ptsd.va.gov

Widom, C. S., Czaja, S. J., & Dutton, M. A. (2008). Childhood victimization and lifetime revictimization. *Child Abuse & Neglect, 32*(8), 785–796. doi:10.1016/j.chiabu.2007.12.006

Zucker, T. L., Samuelson, K. W., Muench, F., Greenberg, M. A., & Gevirtz, R. N. (2009). The effects of respiratory sinus arrhythmia biofeedback on heart rate variability and posttraumatic stress disorder symptoms: A pilot study. *Applied Psychophysiology and Biofeedback, 34*(2), 135. doi:10.1007/s10484-009-9085-2

Supplemental Materials

Table S1
Sample Characteristics

Variable	N = 63 (%)	M(SD)
Age		33.10 (10.01)
Ethnicity (Not Mutually Exclusive)		
White or Caucasian	18 (28.6)	
African American	17 (27.0)	
Hispanic or Latino	13 (20.6)	
Asian	10 (15.9)	
Mixed Race	8 (12.7)	
Black, Non-American	6 (9.5)	
Indian (from India)	3 (4.8)	
Other	4 (6.3)	
Childhood IPV Types Endorsed		
None	19 (30.2)	
Sexual Abuse	24 (38.1)	
Physical Abuse	29 (46.0)	
Emotional Abuse	33 (52.4)	
Polyvictimization Groups		
Type One IPV	15 (23.8)	
Type Two IPV	16 (25.4)	
Type Three IPV	13 (20.6)	

Note. Abbreviations: SD = standard deviation, IPV = interpersonal victimization.

Table S2
Mean Normed Valence and Arousal Ratings for Dot-Probe Stimuli

	Valence		Arousal	
	M	SD	M	SD
High Threat	2.01	(.49)	6.63	(.99)
Mild Threat	3.24	(.86)	5.23	(.79)
Neutral	5.00	(.20)	2.93	(.64)
Positive	7.70	(.51)	4.52	(1.35)

Table S3

IAPS Stimuli Codes by Condition

High Threat	Mild Threat	Positive	Neutral
3000	1270	2158	5500
3030	2900	2530	5520
3181	6190	5760	5531
6313	9630	5833	5534
6350	9920	7470	5535
			7000
			7001
			7002
			7003
			7004
			7006
			7009
			7010
			7012
			7014
			7016
			7017
			7018
			7019
			7045
			7050
			7055
			7056
			7062
			7080
			7090
			7175
			7185
			7187

Note. Numeric codes refer to pictures selected from the International Affective Picture System (IAPS; Lang, Bradley, & Cuthbert, 1999).

Table S4
Correlations of Trauma History and Symptoms by Attention Data

	HT Bias	MT Bias	Pos Bias	HT Diseng	MT Diseng	Pos Diseng	HT RT	MT RT	Pos RT	Neut RT
CTQ Emotional Abuse	-.14	.16	.00	-.10	.11	-.08	-.01	.00	-.02	.00
CTQ Physical Abuse	-.10	.20	.05	-.02	.07	.04	.03	.00	.03	.03
CTQ Sexual Abuse	-.10	.29*	.03	.17	.13	-.06	.24	.16	.17	.19
CTQ Emotional Neglect	-.13	.13	-.01	-.15	.15	-.13	-.07	-.03	-.09	-.04
CTQ Physical Neglect	-.13	.05	.11	-.12	-.09	-.03	-.04	-.05	-.05	-.02
CTQ Total Score	-.15	.23	.04	-.04	.12	-.07	.05	.03	.02	.05
PCL-5 Intrusion	-.03	.35**	.19	.14	.21	.05	.25	.21	.21	.23
PCL-5 Avoidance	.10	.21	.16	.19	.20	.13	.27	.27	.27*	.26*
PCL-5 Neg Mood	.01	.28*	.21	.17	.01	.10	.21	.12	.17	.18
PCL-5 Hyperarousal	-.01	.25*	.13	.10	-.04	-.07	.20	.12	.14	.19
PCL-5 Total	.00	.31*	.19	.16	.08	.05	.24	.18	.20	.22
MDI Disengagement	.11	.05	.17	.13	-.18	-.01	.07	-.02	.01	.05
MDI Depersonalization	-.11	.25*	.15	.10	-.03	-.17	.24	.16	.14	.22
MDI Derealization	.00	.14	.18	.00	-.14	-.06	.07	.02	.03	.09
MDI Emotion Constriction	-.07	.00	.06	-.07	-.26*	-.15	.09	.05	.07	.13
MDI Memory Disturbance	.07	.00	.19	.03	-.25*	-.03	.08	.03	.05	.10
MDI Identity Dissociation	-.02	-.05	.15	-.15	-.18	.03	-.13	-.14	-.12	-.09
MDI Total	.01	.08	.17	.03	-.21	-.09	.10	.03	.05	.11

Note. * Correlation is significant at the 0.05 level (2-tailed). ** Correlation is significant at the 0.01 level (2-tailed).
Abbreviations: CTQ = Childhood Trauma Questionnaire, PCL-5 = PTSD Checklist for DSM 5, MDI = Multiscale Dissociation Inventory, HT = high-threat, MT = mild-threat, Pos = positive, Neut = Neutral, Diseng = disengage, RT = reaction time.

Table S5
Partial Correlations Between Dissociation and Attention, Controlling for PCL-5 PTSD Symptoms

	HT RT	MT RT	Pos RT	Neut RT	HT bias	MT bias	Pos bias	Diseng HT	Diseng MT	Diseng Pos
MDI Disengagement	-.16	-.21†	-.21	-.17	.16	-.27*	.04	.01	-.34**	-.07
MDI Depersonalization	.13	.08	.03	.13	-.14	.10	.05	.01	-.09	-.24
MDI Derealization	-.13	-.15	-.15	-.09	.00	-.11	.07	-.16	-.27*	-.13
MDI Emotion Constriction	-.08	-.08	-.08	-.02	-.10	-.26*	-.08	-.23	-.40**	-.24†
MDI Memory Disturbance	-.11	-.12	-.12	-.07	.09	-.29*	.09	-.11	-.41**	-.09
MDI Identity Dissociation	-.25	-.23†	-.22†	-.20	-.03	-.19	.08	-.24	-.23†	.01
MDI Total	-.12	-.15	-.16	-.08	.00	-.23†	.04	-.14	-.40**	-.18

Note. Abbreviations: MDI = Multiscale Dissociation Inventory, PCL-5 = PTSD Checklist for DSM 5, HT = high-threat, MT = mild-threat, Pos = positive, Diseng = disengage, RT = reaction time
* Correlation is significant at the 0.05 level (2-tailed). ** Correlation is significant at the 0.01 level (2-tailed). † Correlation is marginally significant at the 0.10 level (2-tailed).

6 Digital poly-victimization

The increasing importance of online crime and harassment to the burden of victimization

*Sherry Hamby, Zach Blount, Alli Smith, Lisa Jones,
Kimberly Mitchell, and Elizabeth Taylor*

ABSTRACT

Many forms of victimization, including bullying and property crime, are increasingly moving online, but most studies of poly-victimization still primarily focus on in-person crime and violence. Few studies have examined the importance of incorporating technology-based victimizations for assessing the true burden of violence. The purpose of this study is to explore whether digital poly-victimization contributes to post-traumatic stress and anxiety/dysphoria symptoms after controlling for in-person poly-victimization. Given that technology use and technology-based victimization are changing rapidly, a mixed methods approach was adopted. In the first two phases, focus groups and cognitive interviews (89 total participants) were used to identify the range of digital victimization and develop the Digital Poly-Victimization Scale. In the third phase, the new measure was included in a community survey (n = 478, 57.5% female; 62.6% earning under $50,000 per year) in a rural Southern region, along with measures of in-person poly-victimization, posttraumatic stress and anxiety/dysphoria symptoms, and other outcomes and personal characteristics. A comprehensive measure of digital poly-victimization indicated that almost 3 in 4 participants (72.3%) had experienced at least one form of digital victimization. The results indicated that digital poly-victimization contributed unique variance to post-traumatic stress and anxiety/dysphoria symptoms (*p* < .001), health-related quality of life (*p* < .01), and subjective and family well-being (both *p* < .001), even after controlling for demographics and in-person poly-victimization. Digital victimization often presents fewer risks to perpetrators and can be expected to represent an increasing share of the societal burden of violence. Future research on poly-victimization should pay more attention to the role of digital victimization.

More and more crime is moving online. This should not be particularly surprising, because, from the perpetrator's point of view, there are many advantages to technology-based, or digital, crime. A victim of in-person mugging or bullying might fight back, potentially injuring the perpetrator. There are fewer inhibitory mechanisms in place. Animal aggression, including human aggression, has historically been controlled by a wide range of behavioral cues (Hamby, 2017; Natarajan & Caramaschi, 2010). The digital environment—whether it be cell phones, websites, community gaming sites, or other settings—removes many of the cues that humans, as mammals, have historically also relied on to inhibit aggression. In other words, many people "troll" or "flame" or otherwise say things online or over text that they would not say to a person that is right in front of them (Suler, 2004).

Digital victimization can be defined as victimization (which are intentional, unwanted, nonessential, and harmful experiences, Hamby, 2017) that is perpetrated with the assistance of computerized technology, such as desktops, the Internet, or cell phones. Several new terms for online victimization and related risky behaviors have been coined to capture these emerging phenomena, including "cyberbullying," "sexting," and "phishing" (Jagatic, Johnson, Jakobsson, & Menczer, 2007; Mitchell, Finkelhor, Jones, & Wolak, 2012; Mitchell & Jones, 2015). Based on the most recently available data at the time of writing, 88% of U.S. adults use the Internet, and 77% use a smart phone (Pew Research Center, 2017), which means that vulnerability to digital or "cyber" victimization is nearly as universal as vulnerability to in-person victimization.

The high rates of digital victimization are well known (Anderson, 2006; Internet Crime Complaint, 2014; Reyns, 2013; C. Smith & Agarwal, 2010). The best estimates indicate that approximately 2 out of 5 people in the United States have been affected by cyberbullying and online harassment, which does not even include identity thefts, scams, hacking of accounts, and other financially motivated victimizations (Duggan, 2017). The adverse impact of cyberbullying and online harassment is also well established (e.g., Kowalski & Limber, 2013). The data are especially clear that cyberbullying is associated with trauma symptoms and other adverse outcomes (Hinduja & Patchin, 2010; Staude-Müller, Hansen, & Voss, 2012).

Less is known about financially motivated cyber-victimizations, but existing data suggest that these victimizations are associated with higher levels of psychological distress and other adverse impacts, with some victims falling within the clinical range of depression and anxiety. Although a few items on financial loss have been embedded in longer surveys on online victimization (González & Orgaz, 2014; Mitchell, Sabina, Finkelhor, & Wells, 2009), they have often been combined with safety practices, general use patterns, and other elements that are not related to victimization. A comprehensive assessment of the full range of different types of digital victimization has been lacking.

Another key limitation of existing knowledge is that digital victimization research has been relatively siloed. For example, research on cyberbullying is often conducted independently of other research on in-person bullying (e.g., P. K. Smith et al., 2006). This is true even though studies have indicated it is often the same children involved in-person and online bullying (Mitchell & Jones, 2015; Mitchell, Jones, Turner, Shattuck, & Wolak, 2016).

Poly-victimization and digital crime

Even more significantly, digital victimization has only been partly integrated into the poly-victimization model. Poly-victimization refers to the cumulative burden of the number of different types of victimization experiences. Poly-victimization research has shown that it is the cumulative dose of victimization, more than any one type, that is chiefly responsible for trauma symptoms and other adverse impacts (Ford, Elhai, Connor, & Frueh, 2010; Ford, Grasso, Hawke, & Chapman, 2013; Hamby & Grych, 2013). This research is also consistent with other work on cumulative trauma, such as work on adverse childhood experiences (Felitti et al., 1998).

However, digital victimization has not been well captured in previous work on poly-victimization and cumulative trauma, potentially missing many common victimization experiences in the estimates of total burden. Many commonly used trauma measures do not include digital victimization at all, such as the adverse childhood experiences scale and the Childhood Trauma Questionnaire (Bernstein, Ahluvalia, Pogge, & Handelsman, 1997; Felitti et al., 1998). The National Survey of Children's Exposure to Violence only included two types of digital victimization, general and sexual harassment from online messages, leaving out identity theft and many other types of victimization (Finkelhor, Turner, Ormrod, Hamby, & Kracke, 2009). The item on unwanted sexual messages, while important, is also relatively rare and thus does not well capture the full burden of online victimization. Although the limitations of these measures are due in part to the era when they were created, their unmodified use in the digital age makes their coverage increasingly limited.

Even today, most research on digital victimization, and indeed on crime more generally, pays insufficient attention to digital property crime, including identity theft and financially motivated fraud (Tcherni, Davies, Lopes, & Lizotte, 2016). Property crime is distressing (Plass, 2014). Prior work on poly-victimization shows that conventional theft and vandalism add to the total burden of victimization (Finkelhor, Ormrod, Turner, & Hamby, 2005). Unlike many forms of in-person property crime, which often do not involve a direct confrontation with the victim (Hamby, 2017), many digital forms of property crime involve cons that involve deceiving the victim, sometimes even over long periods of time, such as the "catfishing" con that involves tricking someone into thinking the perpetrator has a sincere romantic interest. Stealing elements of people's identities may also be a particularly upsetting form of property crime, versus stealing cash or electronics or other less personal or sentimental items. The financial costs of online property crime can outstrip in-person thefts (Tcherni et al.,

2016). However, as far as we are aware, no prior studies have examined these sorts of crime in a poly-victimization framework.

The current study

One challenge of research on digital victimization is the rapidly changing technology environment. Some measures refer to America Online, chat rooms, instant messaging, or other already-dated references (Hinduja & Patchin, 2010; P. K. Smith et al., 2008). Even references to "computers" can sound dated as people increasingly rely on cellphones and tablets for all of their computing needs. Thus, this study adopted a mixed-methods approach to capture current experiences, utilizing two phases of qualitative investigation into current digital use and victimization experiences, followed by a large community survey using items developed from the qualitative work. One major goal of the study was also to move beyond cyberbullying and incorporate digital property victimization and "imposter scams" (Federal Trade Commission, 2017) into a comprehensive assessment of adverse digital experiences. Another goal of the study was to examine multiple outcome variables, including post-traumatic stress and anxiety/dysphoria symptoms and other indicators of health, to explore the full impact of victimization. Consistent with the poly-victimization framework (Hamby & Grych, 2013), we anticipate that in-person and digital victimization will be linked. We also hypothesized that digital poly-victimization would explain unique variance in post-traumatic stress and anxiety/dysphoria symptoms and other outcomes, after controlling for in-person poly-victimization.

Method

Participants

The qualitative phases of measurement development of digital victimization consisted of 9 focus groups (4 teen groups and 4 adult groups with 65 total participants; 58% female; 92% White/European American, 3% Latino, 3% multiracial, and 2% African-American) and 24 in-depth individual interviews (25% aged 12–17, 54.2% aged 18–59, 20.8% age 60 or over; 62.5% female; 87.5% White/European American, 8.3% Latino, 4.2% African American). All participants were from the rural southeastern United States, in counties designated as Appalachian by the Appalachian Regional Commission.

The survey included 478 participants from the rural southeastern United States aged 12 to 75 years ($M = 36.44$, $SD = 17.61$) who completed a broader survey on digital online privacy and security and character development. The sample was 57.5% female and 42.5% male; most (84.9%) of the sample identified as White/European American (non-Latino), 5.7% as African American/Black (non-Latino), 4.0% as more than one race, 3.6% as Latino/Latina (any race), .8% as Asian (non-

Latino), and .8% American Indian/Alaska Native (non-Latino). Almost a third of survey participants (29.3%) reported an annual income under $20,000 per year, 33.3% reported earning $20,000 to $50,000, and 37.4% reported earning $50,000 or more. Most of the sample (54.6%) lived in rural areas with populations of less than 2,500 people, 32.7% reported living in small towns with a population of 2,500 to 20,000 people, and others (12.7%) lived in more populous areas.

Procedure

Participants were recruited through a range of advertising techniques. For the qualitative phases, participants were recruited through local organizations and word-of-mouth. In the semi-structured focus groups, participants answered questions regarding technology use, problems faced when using technology (scams), and safety practices that protect their privacy. Each focus group participant received a $20 gift card for participation. The procedures for in-depth individual interviews were similar, with the exception that participants were shown a list of items on different types of digital privacy victimization and other issues that were developed from the focus groups by the research team and previously reviewed by 6 external researchers. Interviewees received a $50 gift card for participation. Focus groups and interviews were audiotaped and transcribed. All procedures received IRB approval from the University of the South.

The majority of survey participants (65.7%) were recruited through word-of-mouth. Recruitment at local community events, such as festivals and county fairs, was the second most productive strategy, accounting for 21.3% of participants. The remaining 13% were recruited through various other strategies, such as website advertisement and through local community organizations. This range of recruitment strategies, which resulted in 96% of the sample being recruited through in-person techniques, allowed us to reach segments of the population who are rarely included in psychological research, including those with limited Internet experience. Technical problems and time limitations at events kept some individuals from completing the survey. The overall completion rate was 94%. The survey was administered as a computer-assisted self-interview, using the Snap11 software platform on computer tablets. On average, the survey took 31 minutes to complete, and each participant received a $20 Walmart gift card and was provided with information on local community resources. Informed consent, including parental consent for minors, was obtained for all participants. All procedures were IRB approved.

Measures

Digital Victimization Scale
The Digital Victimization Scale (Hamby, Smith, & Taylor, 2017) consists of 11 items on a range of online or cellphone-based adverse experiences, including

cyberbullying and cyber-theft of information or money. The items were developed through a three-stage mixed methods process, with the most common and salient experiences first identified in focus groups, then vetted in the individual in-depth interviews, and then revised and incorporated into the survey. The qualitative phase of measurement development yielded a wide range of adverse experiences, including hacking ("[My husband] got hacked three times in a period of six weeks all the way from Florida to Canada."), scams ("I had a friend of mine that got caught in a scam and it was because they thought their friend was in trouble."), using log-ins without permission ("[Son's name] will catch me when I step away from the computer… and he put something [obscene] on … Facebook"), and posting unwanted material ("Someone in my class posted a photo of a teacher, like a weird caption and it was offensive … they got suspended"). We used these to develop a range of items that addressed cyberbullying and related interpersonal harassment as well as financially motivated victimizations.

Dichotomous items ("yes" or "no") were summed to create a digital poly-victimization score. The internal consistency (Cronbach's Alpha) is .70 (inspection of items indicated removing no item would improve the alpha), and in this sample, convergent validity was supported with the bivariate correlation with post-traumatic stress and anxiety/dysphoria, which was symptoms was .31. See Appendix 1 for complete wording.

In-person poly-victimization was assessed with the *Juvenile Victimization Questionnaire—Key Domains Form*, which includes 13 items assessing lifetime history of a range of different types of interpersonal victimization, focusing on childhood victimization experiences such as bullying, child abuse, and exposure to domestic violence (validated in Banyard, Hamby, & Grych, 2017) and adapted from Hamby, Finkelhor, Ormrod, & Turner, 2004. A sample item is "During your childhood, did one of your parents get hit or pushed by another parent?" Dichotomous items ("yes" or "no") were summed to create an in-person poly-victimization score. Cronbach's Alpha was .84, and in this sample convergent validity was supported with bivariate correlations with digital poly-victimization (.37; $p < .001$) and post-traumatic stress and anxiety/dysphoria symptoms (.34; $p < .001$).

Post-traumatic stress and anxiety/dysphoria symptoms

Eight psychological symptoms associated with post-traumatic stress disorder and other anxiety and mood disorders (adapted from Briere, 1996; Finkelhor et al., 2011 based on the best-performing items in those scales, with simplified language for our sample) were assessed on a 4-point scale from "never" to "almost all the time." A sample item is "Feeling lonely in the last month." Higher scores indicate more post-traumatic stress and anxiety/dysphoria symptoms. Internal consistency (Cronbach's Alpha) was .89, and in this sample, convergent validity was supported with a bivariate correlation of -.29 ($p < .001$)

with Health-Related Quality of Life. Also see Hamby, Grych, & Banyard, 2017 for additional evidence of convergent validity. See Appendix 2 for complete wording.

Health-related quality of life

Five items assessing physical health and well-being were adapted from the "Healthy Days Measure" used by the U.S. Centers for Disease Control and Prevention (CDC, 2000). Items use a 5-point scale measuring frequency in the past 30 days, ranging from "0 days" to "Every day or almost every day." Another item assessed self-reported general health on a 5-point scale, ranging from "poor" to "excellent," with higher scores indicated higher health-related quality of life. A sample item is, "During the past 30 days, how many days was your physical health, which includes physical illness and injury, not good?" Internal consistency (Cronbach's Alpha) was .79, and in this sample, convergent validity was supported with bivariate correlations with Subjective Well-Being (.34; $p < .001$) and Family Well-Being (.28; $p < .001$) (also see Hamby et al., 2017).

Subjective well-being (Hamby, Banyard, Grych, Smith, & Taylor, 2017)

Four items assessing one's satisfaction with the quality of life were developed using focus group and interview input as well as a review of other measures (Battista & Almond, 1973; Diener, Emmons, Larsen, & Griffin, 1985; Pavot & Diener, 1993; Pearlin & Schooler, 1978; Rosenberg, 1965; Turner et al., 2012). A sample item is "I am happy with myself." Cronbach's Alpha was .87, and in this sample, the bivariate correlation with post-traumatic growth was .52 ($p < .001$) and a -.43 ($p < .001$) correlation with trauma symptoms (for additional validity evidence, see Hamby, Banyard, Grych, Smith, & Taylor, 2017).

Family well-being

Four items assessing the positivity, happiness, and well-being within the family were adapted and modified from the subjective well-being measure (Hamby et al., 2017). Items were scored on a 4-point scale ranging from "not true about my family" to "mostly true about my family," with higher scores indicating higher family well-being. A sample item is, "My family has a lot to be proud of." Cronbach's Alpha was .85, and evidence of convergent validity is the bivariate correlation with Subjective Well-Being was .51 ($p < .001$) (also see Hamby, Blount, Taylor, & Smith, 2017).

Data analysis

As noted in the measures section, the first two qualitative phases were used to develop the Digital Victimization Scale, using content analysis and grounded theory analysis of focus groups and interviews. Descriptive statistics characterized rates of victimization and described the sample. Missing data were very low (0% to 2.3%), except for household income, which was 7.5%, well under the levels recommended by Bennett (2001). Non-demographic data were imputed. Odds ratios were calculated to test whether the experiences of in-person and of digital poly-victimization were related. Hierarchical regression was used to explore the contribution digital poly-victimization experiences to a range of outcomes. In each regression, we first entered age, gender, and household income, and then in the second block, we added poly-victimization. Finally, in the third block, digital poly-victimization was added to see if it made a contribution to psychological or health status after controlling for in-person poly-victimization and demographic variables. We conducted this regression for five different outcome variables: post-traumatic stress and anxiety/dysphoria symptoms, health-related quality of life, subjective well-being, and spiritual well-being.

Results

Rates of in-person and digital poly-victimization

Most of our participants (84%) reported at least one form of in-person victimization during the course of their lifetime, with a mean of 4.03 lifetime victimization types per person (SD = 3.38). Digital victimization was somewhat less common in this sample, but still prevalent. Almost 3 in 4 participants (72.3%) reported at least one digital victimization, with a mean of 1.86 different types of victimization per person (SD = 1.92). Consistent with the poly-victimization framework, participants reporting any in-person victimization were more as likely to also report at least one type of digital victimization, odds ratio = 2.17 (95% confidence interval 1.30–3.60), $p < .01$. Approximately 3 in 4 (74.9%) of in-person victims reported digital victimization, compared to 57.9% of those who had not experienced in-person victimization.

Post-traumatic stress and anxiety/dysphoria symptoms and victimization

In the first block of the hierarchical regression for post-traumatic stress and anxiety/dysphoria symptoms, age and income were both significantly related to symptoms, in the inverse direction (see Table 1). Older participants and those with higher incomes reported fewer symptoms than others. Poly-victimization added significantly more variance, with a change (Δ) in R^2 of 11.1%. As predicted, a higher burden of in-person victimization was associated with higher post-traumatic stress and anxiety/dysphoria symptoms in the past month. Digital poly-victimization, in the third block, added significant additional variance to the equation, although less variance than explained by in-person victimization (change in R^2 of 3% vs 11.1%). Income was no longer significant

Table 1. Hierarchical multiple regression analyses predicting post-traumatic stress and anxiety/dysphoria symptoms.

Predictor	Total R^2	ΔR^2	B	β	CI for B (95%)	
Step 1 ***	.047	.047				
Age			−.058	−.170***	−.091;	−.026
Gender			−.051	−.004	−1.194;	1.092
Household Income			−.985	−.135**	−1.674;	−.297
Step 2 ***	.158	.111				
Age			−.069	−.202***	−.100;	−.039
Gender			.212	.018	−.866;	1.290
Household Income			−.664	−.091*	−1.318;	−.011
Poly-victimization			.593	.337***	.437;	.749
Step 3 ***	.188	.030				
Age			−.068	−.198***	−.098;	−.038
Gender			.313	.026	−.748;	1.374
Household Income			−.590	−.081	−1.233;	.054
Poly-victimization			.474	.269***	.310;	.638
Digital Poly-victimization			.601	.188***	.304;	.897
Total R^2 for full model	.188					

***p < .001, **p < .01, *p < .05. ΔR^2 = change in percent of variance explained at each step.

after controlling for digital poly-victimization. The total R^2 for the full model including all variables was 18.8%.

Health-related quality of life and victimization

In Block 1 of this hierarchical regression, age was inversely associated with health-related quality of life, while household income was positively associated with this outcome variable. Younger participants and those with higher household incomes reported higher health-related quality of life. Poly-victimization was also inversely associated with health-related quality of life in the second block, adding significantly more variance to the equation (ΔR^2 = 4.8%). In the third block, digital poly-victimization also added significantly more variance (ΔR^2 = 2.1%), with participants experiencing more digital victimization also reporting lower levels of health quality. In the third block, age, household income, and poly-victimization all remained significant. The full equation accounted for 20.1% of the variance in health-related quality of life. See Table 2 for regression results.

Subjective well-being and victimization

For subjective well-being, household income was positively associated with subjective well-being in the first block, but age and gender were not significant. In the second block, poly-victimization added significant additional variance to the equation (ΔR^2 = 3.7%) and was inversely associated with subjective well-being. Digital poly-victimization added significant variance in the third block

Table 2. Hierarchical multiple regression analyses predicting health-related quality of life.

Predictor	Total R^2	ΔR^2	B	β	CI for B (95%)	
Step 1 ***	.132	.132				
Age			−.047	−.191***	−.070;	−.025
Gender			−.028	−.003	−.814;	.758
Household Income			1.614	.306***	1.140;	2.088
Step 2 ***	.180	.048				
Age			−.042	−.170***	−.064;	−.020
Gender			−.156	−.018	−.922;	.611
Household Income			1.462	.278***	−.997;	1.927
Poly-victimization			−.282	−.222***	−.393;	−.171
Step 3 **	.201	.021				
Age			−.043	−.174***	−.065;	−.021
Gender			−.217	−.025	−.976;	.542
Household Income			1.417	.269***	.957;	1.878
Poly-victimization			−.211	−.166***	−.328;	−.093
Digital Poly-victimization			−.358	−.155**	−.570;	−.146
Total R^2 for full model	.201					

***$p < .001$, **$p < .01$, *$p < .05$. ΔR^2 = change in percent of variance explained at each step.

Table 3. Hierarchical multiple regression analyses predicting subjective well-being.

Predictor	Total R^2	ΔR^2	B	β	CI for B (95%)	
Step 1 **	.031	.031				
Age			.008	.056	−.006;	.023
Gender			.307	.059	−.194;	.809
Household Income			.518	.163**	.215;	.820
Step 2 ***	.068	.037				
Age			.011	.074	−.003;	.025
Gender			.238	.046	−.255;	.732
Household Income			.440	.138**	.140;	.739
Poly-victimization			−.148	−.194***	−.220;	−.077
Step 3 ***	.107	.039				
Age			.010	.069	−.003;	.024
Gender			.189	.036	−.296;	.673
Household Income			.401	.126**	.107;	.694
Poly-victimization			−.089	−.117*	−.164;	−.015
Digital Poly-victimization			−.298	−.214***	−.434;	−.163
Total R^2 for full model	.107					

***$p < .001$, **$p < .01$, *$p < .05$. ΔR^2 = change in percent of variance explained at each step.

($\Delta R^2 = 3.9\%$; total $R^2 = 10.7\%$), with more digital poly-victimization associated with lower subjective well-being. Household income and poly-victimization remained positively and negatively associated with subjective well-being, respectively. See Table 3 for regression results.

Family well-being and victimization

For family well-being, household income was positively related to family well-being in the first block, but age and gender were not significant. Poly-victimization added significantly more variance ($\Delta R^2 = 7.8\%$), and as

Table 4. Hierarchical multiple regression analyses predicting family well-being.

Predictor	Total R^2	ΔR^2	B	β	CI for B (95%)	
				Outcome: Family Well-Being		
Step 1 **	.038	.038				
Age			−.005	−.034	−.018;	.009
Gender			.167	.034	−.301;	.634
Household Income			.584	.197***	.302;	.866
Step 2 ***	.116	.078				
Age			−.001	−.007	−.014;	.012
Gender			.073	.015	−.377;	.523
Household Income			.479	.161**	.207;	.752
Poly-victimization			−.202	−.282***	−.267;	−.137
Step 3 ***	.151	.035				
Age			−.002	−.011	−.014;	.011
Gender			.027	.006	−.415;	.469
Household Income			.447	.151**	.179;	.715
Poly-victimization			−.150	−.210***	−.219;	−.082
Digital Poly-victimization			−.262	−.201***	−.385;	−.138
Total R^2 for full model	.151					

***$p < .001$, **$p < .01$, *$p < .05$. ΔR^2 = change in percent of variance explained at each step.

predicted, poly-victimization was associated with lower family well-being. In the third block, digital poly-victimization also added significant variance ($\Delta R^2 = 3.5\%$) and was inversely associated with family well-being, resulting in a total R^2 of 15.1%. Household income remained positively associated, and poly-victimization remained inversely associated with family well-being in the third block. See Table 4 for regression results.

Discussion

In this community sample, digital poly-victimization is a significant component of the true burden of victimization. Analyses indicated that digital poly-victimization contributed unique variance to post-traumatic stress and anxiety/dysphoria symptoms and three other outcome variables, even after controlling for in-person poly-victimization and demographic characteristics. This was largely consistent with predictions. Digital victimization (mono- or poly-victimization) was also a prevalent experience, with almost 3 in 4 respondents reporting at least one type of digital victimization experience. Qualitative data also supported the premise that there are a wide range of types of digital victimization that people experience. Also consistent with predictions, those with an in-person victimization history were more likely to experience at least one digital victimization than those who reported no in-person victimizations (74.9% versus 57.9%). As more crime moves online, it will become increasingly important to recognize the impact of digital poly-victimization, including not only cyberbullying but other widespread forms of digital victimization, such as online fraud and identity theft (Tcherni et al., 2016). A comparison of the bivariate and multivariate analyses suggests that some of the variance in post-traumatic stress and anxiety/dysphoria symptoms is similar for in-person and digital victimization. The bivariate correlations with post-traumatic stress and anxiety/dysphoria symptoms were similar for both scales (.31 and .34). However, the multivariate results indicate that digital victimization has a unique impact beyond the more typically measured in-person victimization. This is consistent with current thinking on poly-victimization, which suggests that the number of distinct violations—especially different settings and different perpe-trators— has the largest impact on post-traumatic stress and anxiety/dysphoria symptoms. As more of our interactions move online, it is important that research captures this domain where vulnerability is high. As far as we are aware, this is the first study to show that digital poly-victimization is uniquely associated with post-traumatic stress and anxiety/dysphoria symptoms and other outcomes.

The finding that digital poly-victimization is adding significantly to individuals' victimization burdens is largely consistent with more siloed research on the burden of online crime (Jones, Mitchell, & Finkelhor, 2012; Kowalski & Limber, 2013). Some have even suggested that the much-vaunted reduction in crime could be eliminated if a full reckoning of digital victimi-zation was included in crime rates (Tcherni et al., 2016). The high rates of reporting both in-person and online victimization are also consistent with research indicating that, like other research into the web of violence (Hamby & Grych, 2013), many people are being victimized via both modalities (Mitchell & Jones, 2015).

This study also adds to the limited evidence base of the digital victimization experiences of rural, low-income residents. Although some people with lower incomes have less technology experience (A. Smith, 2013), it is a misconception that people living in a rural area would not be apt to experience any digital victimization. Our study demonstrates that people in rural residences experience digital poly-victimization at high rates and that it contributes to their overall burden of victimization. Rural and low-income populations should not be excluded from studies involving digital poly-victimization; it is our hope that future studies will work to develop prevention efforts to combat digital poly-victimization in all populations.

Strengths and limitations

The results of this study should be considered in light of the strengths and limitations of the project. To our knowledge, this is the first study to examine the unique contribution of digital poly-victimization, beyond in-person poly-victimization, on post-traumatic stress and anxiety/dysphoria symptoms and a variety of other outcome measures. It is also one of the few to study online victimization in residents of rural Appalachia. Appalachia, one of the largest low-income regions of the United States, is an under-studied region that can be hard to access for outsiders (Woodard, 2011), and our large community sample from this area is a strength. However, at the same time, the region has unique demographic characteristics, such as below average income relative to the rest of the United States and less racial and ethnic diversity than many regions of the country. Although we believe our sampling strategy effectively recruited many people who seldom participate in survey research, the non-random sample may have unknown biases. This was a cross-sectional study, which is an appropriate and cost-effective means of exploring new ideas, but would benefit from replication in a longitudinal study. It included a broad range of ages, from adolescence through adulthood. The creation and adaptation of numerous strengths measures in the context of digital-poly-victimization for a low-income community sample involving youth as young as age 12 also is a strength. Though not included in our version of digital victimization, malicious sexting should also be addressed by future research. Prior work has found that sexting is considered a risky behavior, and when sexting coercion is involved, it has been found to have a negative impact on mental health (Mitchell et al., 2012; Ross, Drouin, & Coupe, 2016). It would be worthwhile for future research to investigate the recency and severity of digital victimization as possible factors affecting the impact. Further research is needed to determine whether specific types of digital victimization are responsible for its association with distress (as opposed to the cumulative score used in these analyses).

Research and clinical implications

As patterns of crime change due to the growing prevalence of Internet and online activities, researchers and clinicians should enhance their assessment tools in order to provide coverage of issues regarding digital poly-victimization. Most immediately, we encourage professionals to add questions on digital experiences to any assessment of victimization, and to further explore the links between in-person and digital poly-victimization. Clinicians should be aware that digital victimization is a common experience that has probably affected many of their clients, at least as mono-victims and in many cases as poly-victims too. Any assessment should include the full range of types of digital victimization, including financially motivated victimizations as well as interpersonal offenses, in order to adequately capture the true burden of victimization. Measures that are limited to cyberbullying are not sufficiently capturing digital poly-victimization. Our estimates of digital poly-victimization are almost twice as high as recent estimates based primarily on cyberbullying and harassment (Duggan, 2017)

Regarding prevention and intervention, there are many efforts to teach "media" skills regarding fake news and other challenges. We should be teaching youth and other less experienced computer users basic skills in recognizing cons and frauds. Although we did not directly assess fraud attempts that did not lead to victimization, based on our own experiences, we assume that this is a regular experience for most individuals. Skills in navigating fraudulent offers is a new basic skill that should be required content in schools and in violence prevention programming. As more and more of our daily interactions migrate to online and other digital modalities, it is essential that violence research, prevention, and intervention keep pace with these social changes.

Funding

This research was supported by the Digital Trust Foundation. The opinions in this paper do not necessarily represent the opinions of the Digital Trust Foundation.We thank the participants of our study for helping us to understand digital victimization.

References

Anderson, K. (2006). Who are the victims of identity theft? The effect of demographics. *Journal of Public Policy & Marketing, 25*(2), 160–171.

Banyard, V., Hamby, S., & Grych, J. (2017). Health effects of adverse childhood events: Identifying promising protective factors at the intersection of mental and physical well-being. *Child Abuse & Neglect, 65,* 88–98.

Battista, J., & Almond, R. (1973). The development of meaning in life. *Psychiatry, 36*(4), 409–427.

Bennett, D. A. (2001). How can I deal with missing data in my study? *Australian and New Zealand Journal of Public Health, 25*(5), 464–469.

Bernstein, D. P., Ahluvalia, T., Pogge, D., & Handelsman, L. (1997). Validity of the childhood trauma questionnaire in an adolescent psychiatric population. *Journal of the American Academy of Child & Adolescent Psychiatry, 36*(3), 340–348.

Briere, J. (1996). *Trauma Symptoms Checklist for Children (TSCC): Professional manual.* Odessa, FL: Psychological Assessent Resources.

CDC, C. F. D. C. A. P. (2000). *Measuring healthy days: Population assessment of health-related quality of life.* Retrieved from: http://www.cdc.gov/hrqol/pdfs/mhd.pdf

Diener, E., Emmons, R., Larsen, R., & Griffin, S. (1985). The satisfaction with life scale. *Journal of Personality Assessment, 49*(1), 71–75.

Duggan, M. (2017). *Online harassment.* Washington, DC: Pew Research Center. Retrieved from http://assets.pewresearch.org/wp-content/uploads/sites/14/2017/07/10151519/PI_2017.07.11_Online-Harassment_FINAL.pdf

Federal Trade Commission. (2017). *Consumer sentinel network data book for January - December 2016.* Retrieved from https://www.ftc.gov/system/files/documents/reports/consumer-sentinel-network-data-book-january-december-2016/csn_cy-2016_data_book.pdf

Felitti, V. J., Anda, R. F., Nordenberg, D., Williamson, D. F., Spitz, A. M., Edwards, V., … Marks, J. S. (1998). Relationship of childhood abuse and household dysfunction to many of the leading causes of death in adults: The adverse childhood experiences (ACE) study. *American Journal of Preventative Medicine, 14*(4), 245–258.

Finkelhor, D., Ormrod, R. K., Turner, H. A., & Hamby, S. L. (2005). Measuring poly-victimization using the juvenile victimization questionnaire. *Child Abuse & Neglect, 29*(11), 1297–1312.

Finkelhor, D., Turner, H., Hamby, S.L., & Ormrod, R. (2011). *Polyvictimization: Children's exposure to multiple types of violence, crime, and abuse.* Washington, DC: Office of Juvenile Justice and Delinquency Prevention, U.S. Department of Justice.

Finkelhor, D., Turner, H., Ormrod, R., Hamby, S., & Kracke, K. (2009). *Children's exposure to violence: A comprehensive national survey.*Bulletin. Washington, DC: U.S. Department of Justice, Office of Justice Programs, Office of Juvenile Justice and Delinquency Prevention.

Ford, J. D., Elhai, J. D., Connor, D. F., & Frueh, C. (2010). Poly-victimization and risk of posttraumatic, depressive, and substance use disorders and involvement in delinquency in a national sample of adolescents. *Journal of Adolescent Health, 46,* 545–552. doi:10.1016/j.jadohealth.2009.11.212

Ford, J. D., Grasso, D. J., Hawke, J., & Chapman, J. F. (2013). Poly-victimization among juvenile justice-involved youths. *Child Abuse & Neglect, 37*(10), 788–800.

González, E., & Orgaz, B. (2014). Problematic online experiences among Spanish college students: Associations with internet use characteristics and clinical symptoms. *Computers in Human Behavior, 31,* 151–158. doi:10.1016/j.chb.2013.10.038

Hamby, S. (2017). On defining violence, and why it matters. *Psychology of Violence, 7*(2), 167–180.

Hamby, S., Banyard, V., Grych, J., Smith, A., & Taylor, E. (2017). *Subjective well-being scale.* Monteagle, TN: Life Paths Appalachian Research Center.

Hamby, S., Blount, Z., Taylor, E., & Smith, A. (2017). *Family well-being scale.* Monteagle, TN: Life Paths Appalachian Research Center.

Hamby, S., Finkelhor, D., Ormrod, R. K., & Turner, H. A. (2004). *The juvenile victimization questionnaire (JVQ): Administration and scoring manual.* Durham, NH: Crimes Against Children Research Center.

Hamby, S., & Grych, J. (2013). *The web of violence: Exploring connections among forms of interpersonal violence and abuse.* New York, NY: Springer.

Hamby, S., Grych, J., & Banyard, V. (2017). Resilience portfolios and poly-strengths: Identifying protective factors associated with thriving after adversity. *Psychology of Violence.* Advanced online publication.

Hamby, S., Smith, A., & Taylor, E. (2017). *Digital poly-victimization scale.* Monteagle, TN: Life Paths Appalachian Research Center.

Hinduja, S., & Patchin, J. W. (2010). Bullying, cyberbullying, and suicide. *Archives of Suicide Research, 14*(3), 206–221. doi:10.1080/13811118.2010.494133

Internet Crime Complaint Center. (2014). *2014 Internet crime report.* Retrieved from https://www.fbi.gov/news/news_blog/2014-ic3-annual-report

Jagatic, T. N., Johnson, N. A., Jakobsson, M., & Menczer, F. (2007). Social phishing. *Communications of the ACM, 50*(10), 94–100.

Jones, L., Mitchell, K., & Finkelhor, D. (2012). Trends in youth internet victimization: Findings from three youth internet safety surveys 2000-2010. *Journal of Adolescent Health, 50*(2), 179–186.

Kowalski, R. M., & Limber, S. P. (2013). Psychological, physical, and academic correlates of cyberbullying and traditional bullying. *Journal of Adolescent Health, 53,* S13–S20. doi:10.1016/j.jadohealth.2012.09.018

Mitchell, K., Finkelhor, D., Jones, L., & Wolak, J. (2012). Prevalence and characteristics of youth sexting: A national study. *Pediatrics, 129*(1), 13–20.

Mitchell, K., Jones, L., Turner, H., Shattuck, A., & Wolak, J. (2016). The role of technology in peer harassment: does it amplify harm for youth? *Psychology of Violence, 6*(2), 193–204. doi:10.1037/a0039317

Mitchell, K., & Jones, L. M. (2015). Cyberbullying and bullying must be studied within a broader peer victimization framework. *Journal of Adolescent Health, 56,* 473–474. doi:10.1016/j.jadohealth.2015.02.005

Mitchell, K., Sabina, C., Finkelhor, D., & Wells, M. (2009). Index of problematic online experiences: Item characteristics and correlation with negative symptomatology. *Cyberpsychology & Behavior, 12*(6), 707–711.

Natarajan, D., & Caramaschi, D. (2010). Animal violence demystified. *Frontiers in Behavioral Neuroscience, 4*(9), 1–16.

Pavot, W., & Diener, E. (1993). Review of the satisfaction with life scale. *Psychological Assessment, 5*(2), 164–172.

Pearlin, L., & Schooler, C. (1978). The structure of coping. *Journal of Health & Social Behavior, 19,* 2–21.

Pew Research Center. (2017). Internet/Broadband fact sheet. Retrieved from http://www.pewinternet.org/fact-sheet/internet-broadband/

Plass, P. S. (2014). Property crime victimizations in childhood: A retrospective study. *Journal of Human Behavior in the Social Environment, 24*(4), 448–461.

Reyns, B. (2013). Online routine and identity theft victimization: Further expanding routine activity theory beyond direct-contact offenses. *Journal of Research in Crime & Deliquency, 50*(2), 216–238.

Rosenberg, M. (1965). *Society and the adolescent self-image.* Princeton, NJ: Princeton University Press.

Ross, J. M., Drouin, M., & Coupe, A. (2016). Sexting coercion as a component of intimate partner polyvictimization. *Journal of Interpersonal Violence.* doi:10.1177/0886260516660300

Smith, A. (2013). *Technology adoption by lower income populations.* Retrieved from http://www.pewinternet.org/files/old-media/Files/Presentations/2013/APHSA%20Aaron%20Smith%20Presentation_PDF.pdf

Smith, C., & Agarwal, R. (2010). Practicing safe computing: A multimedia empirical examination of home computer user security behavioral patterns. *MIS Quarterly, 34*(3), 613–643.

Smith, P., Mahdavi, J., Carvalho, M., & Tippett, N. (2006). An investigation into cyberbullying, its forms, awareness and impact, and the relationship between age and gender in cyberbullying (RBX03-06)London: DIES.

Smith, P. K., Mahdavi, J., Carvalho, M., Fisher, S., Russell, S., & Tippett, N. (2008). Cyberbullying: Its nature and impact in secondary school pupils. *The Journal of Child Psychology and Psychiatry, 49*(4), 376–385. doi:10.1111/j.1469-7610.2007.01846.x

Staude-Müller, F., Hansen, B., & Voss, M. (2012). How stressful is online victimization? Effects of victim's personality and properties of the incident. *European Journal of Developmental Psychology, 9*(2), 260–274.

Suler, J. (2004). The online disinhibition effect. *Cyberpsychology & Behavior, 7*(3), 321–326.

Tcherni, M., Davies, A., Lopes, G., & Lizotte, A. (2016). The dark figure of online property crime: Is cyberspace hiding a crime wave? *Justice Quarterly, 33*(5), 890–911.

Turner, H., Finkelhor, D., Ormrod, R. K., Hamby, S., Leeb, R., Mercy, J., & Holt, M. (2012). Family context, victimization, and child trauma symptoms: Variations in safe, stable, and nurturing relationships during early and middle childhood. *American Journal of Orthopsychiatry, 82*(2), 209–219.

Woodard, C. (2011). *American nations: A history of the eleven rival regional cultures of North America*. New York, NY: Penguin.

Appendix 1

Digital Victimization Scale

The next questions ask about people who have contacted you online or on your phone. We mean anyone who contacted you over a phone, email, app, computer, or other device.

1. Someone tricked me into giving personal information over my phone, tablet, or computer.

2. Someone stole information or money from me by "hacking" or breaking into an online account.

3. I have been upset by ads or offers that seem to have personal information about me.

4. I have been upset by the amount of information that I have to share to get apps or programs I need.

5. Someone caused problems for me when they pretended to be me online.

6. Someone caused problems for me when they used my log-in without permission.

7. Someone caused problems for me when they said mean things about me online.

8. Someone caused problems for me when they forwarded embarrassing text messages or pictures.

9. Someone caused problems for me when they tracked my location online.

10. Someone caused problems for me when they told lies or spread rumors about me online.

11. Someone caused problems for me when they kept me out of online groups or group messages.

Note: All items were scored on a two-point scale as either "yes" or "no." Copyright 2017 Sherry Hamby, Elizabeth Taylor, Alli Smith, Zach Blount, Lisa Jones, and Kimberly Mitchell. Reprinted by permission.

Appendix 2

Post-traumatic Stress and Anxiety/Dysphoria Symptoms Scale

These statements describe things that people sometimes think, feel, or do. Please say how true each sentence has been for you in the last month.

1. Feeling lonely in the last month.
2. Feeling sad in the last month.
3. Feeling like shouting at people in the last month.
4. Feeling stupid or like a bad person in the last month.
5. Feeling like I did something wrong in the last month.
6. Feeling worried or anxious in the last month.
7. Trying not to think in the last month.
8. Remembering upsetting or bad things that happened in the last month.

Note: All items were scored on a four-point scale ranging from "never" to "almost all the time." Copyright 2017 Sherry Hamby and Elizabeth Taylor. Reprinted by permission.

Index

Printed and bound by CPI Group (UK) Ltd, Croydon, CR0 4YY

24/10/2024

01778293-0016